2 0 2 2
CDI
POCKET
GUIDE®

Richard D. Pinson, MD, FACP, CCS
and
Cynthia L. Tang, RHIA, CCS, CRC

2022 CDI Pocket Guide® 15th Edition
is published by Pinson & Tang, LLC

Copyright © 2021 Pinson&Tang LLC. Printed in the United States of America

ISBN: 978-1-7334594-4-0

Quantity discounts available. For more information, go to our website or contact:

Pinson & Tang LLC
Houston, Texas
Email: info@pinsonandtang.com

Subscribe to receive important updates, articles, and upcoming webinars at:

www.cdipocketguide.com

The first edition of this guide was born in 2008, after a long gestation period. As a consultant, Cynthia Tang witnessed first-hand the burden of typical CDI training in the 1990s: CDI staff would be given large binders containing hundreds of pages of information, which was difficult to search through and even more difficult to learn from, and the information was proprietary to the large consulting firms. The only way to gain expert knowledge was to be in a hospital that was willing to hire consultants like her to train the staff.

Cynthia envisioned improving both hospital finances and the daily lives of coding and CDI specialists by creating a handy reference guide that would be accessible to all who needed it. She conceived of a pocket-sized book for the CDI staff to use when they visited the nursing units. She felt such a guide needed the imprimatur of a practicing physician, however, and serendipity answered the need in 2006 when she met Dr. Richard Pinson. They shared a desire to create a simple, easy-to-use guide that streamlined information and explained it in a way that everyone could easily understand, all with the goal of helping hospitals and physicians achieve accurate, thorough, and compliant documentation.

So Cynthia and Richard joined forces and started their own consulting firm. Together they wrote the first edition of the *CDI Pocket Guide*, published in 2008. It was an immediate and resounding success with their clients. To achieve a broader reach, they agreed in 2011 to have HCPro/ACDIS publish the book. They decided to self-publish in 2020 to reach an even broader audience, expand their digital editions and reduce its cost, which had been prohibitive for some. The original *CDI Pocket Guide*® remains the best-selling comprehensive CDI resource guide for documentation specialists, coding professionals, and providers.

Other reference guides by Pinson & Tang:
- CDI Pocket Guide® Unbound (on-line) edition
- Outpatient CDI Pocket Guide®: Focusing on HCCs
- CDI Pocket Guide® for ICD-10-AM and AR-DRGs (International edition)

INTRODUCTION TO THE CDI POCKET GUIDE®, 15TH EDITION

We trust that you, like thousands before you, will find this a useful tool in addressing the daily complexities of coding and clinical documentation. The ultimate goal is not just more accurate coding and reimbursement, but improved quality and outcomes for both physician and hospital.

Each of the five sections of this guide is written with a specific purpose in mind:

Guidelines is a shortcut to the most important guidelines and coding rules for DRG assignment and other important topics. Refer to these guidelines frequently.

Key References provides detailed clinical definitions, diagnostic criteria, treatment, coding and documentation challenges, and references for the most important and frequently encountered conditions.

Comorbid Conditions lists and summarizes the most common and important MCC, CC, and HCC conditions with standard SOI subclass that affect MS-DRG/APR-DRG assignment and quality and performance metrics.

DRG Tips includes alternative DRG selection for select DRGs which in our experience have a likelihood of another principal diagnosis, MCC or CC, or procedure.

MS-DRG Table is a complete list of the most recent MS-DRGs, their relative weights, transfer DRG status, and GMLOS for quick reference.

To your success,

Dr. Richard Pinson and Cynthia Tang

The ICD-10-CM and ICD-10-PCS authoritative sources for coding and reporting are listed below. These should be reviewed and referenced routinely for specific situations and circumstances to ensure accurate coding.

1. ICD-10 Coding Classifications
2. Official Coding Guidelines for Coding & Reporting
3. AHA Coding Clinic

The instructions and coding conventions in ICD-10 take **precedence** over the Official Coding Guidelines (OCG), which in turn take precedence over Coding Clinic advice. Coding Clinic advice is the official source of advice where ICD-10 and the OCG are ambiguous, conflicting or silent. Coding Clinic for ICD-10 began in 2012. In the absence of changes to ICD-10 codes and guidance, prior Coding Clinics will stand as long as there is nothing new published by Coding Clinic to replace them.

When there is a **discrepancy** between the conventions in the classification, the guidelines, and/or advice published in Coding Clinic, coding professionals should adhere to the hierarchy shown above. Coding Clinic advises to submit any apparent conflicts with the specific case example(s) and rationale to the AHA Central Office for review.

Excludes Notes. ICD-10-CM defines two types of Excludes notes:

- **Excludes1** means "Not Coded Here." The code excluded should not be used at the same time as the code above the Excludes1 note. The two conditions cannot be coded together, except when the two conditions are clearly unrelated to each other.

- **Excludes2** means "Not Included Here." The condition excluded is not part of the condition it is excluded from, but a patient may have both conditions at the same time. It is acceptable to code both together.

EXAMPLES N39.0 Urinary tract infection, site not specified. Excludes1: Cystitis (N30.-)

D63.0 Anemia in neoplastic disease. Excludes2: Anemia due to antineoplastic chemotherapy (D64.81)

DEFINITION OF THE PRINCIPAL DIAGNOSIS

Official Coding Guidelines (OCG) Section II specifies rules for the selection of the principal diagnosis, first noting that the definition is:

"That condition established after study to be chiefly responsible for occasioning the admission of the patient to the hospital for care."

The words "after study" in the definition are important, since it is not necessarily the admitting diagnosis, but rather the diagnosis found after diagnostic workup (or surgery) that proved to be the primary reason for or focus of the admission.

Consider WHY the patient was admitted to the hospital and could not be in observation or go home. Many patients are admitted with several medical problems, but those that could have been individually treated as an outpatient or observation are unlikely to be chiefly responsible for the admission.

The condition (or at least some signs or symptoms referable to the condition) must have been present on admission. But in some cases, it may be several days before the provider arrives at or documents a definitive diagnosis. This does not mean that the condition was not present on admission if the signs and symptoms of it were present on admission (POA).

The OCG POA Guidelines includes an important definition of POA with implications for assigning the principal diagnosis: Diagnoses subsequently confirmed after admission are considered POA if at the time of admission they *"constitute an underlying cause of a symptom that is present at the time of admission."*

The **circumstances of admission** always govern the selection of the principal diagnosis (unless coding guidance states otherwise), and the selection of the principal diagnosis is based on the entire medical record: *"The entire record should be reviewed to determine the specific reason for the encounter and the conditions treated."* (OCG p. 1).

Important considerations for determining circumstances of admission:

- Severity of each condition or greatest mortality/complication risk
- Complexity of care, evaluation, management
- Medications required, risks, route of administration (IV vs. po)
- Diagnostic procedures, number and types of consultants
- Intensity of monitoring (vital signs, nursing time, etc.)
- Plans for follow-up care

When treatment is totally or primarily directed toward one condition, or only one condition would have required inpatient care, that condition would be designated as principal diagnosis. In most circumstances, the diagnosis for which a major surgical procedure is performed would be assigned as the principal diagnosis. See ***Unrelated OR Procedure DRGs***.

1. TWO OR MORE DIAGNOSES THAT EQUALLY MEET THE CRITERIA FOR PRINCIPAL DIAGNOSIS

"In the unusual instance when two or more diagnoses equally meet the criteria for principal diagnosis as ***determined by the circumstances of admission, diagnostic workup, and/or therapy provided*** and the Alphabetic Index, Tabular List, or another coding guideline does not provide sequencing direction, any one of the diagnoses may be sequenced first." (OCG Section II.C).

It is not uncommon for a patient to be admitted with multiple conditions. When management is equally directed toward more than one condition and each condition would typically require inpatient care, any one of the diagnoses can be assigned as principal diagnosis.

> **EXAMPLES**   Pt admitted with CHF and pneumonia. Pt given IV Lasix and IV antibiotics.
>
> Pt admitted with acute atrial fibrillation and acute heart failure. Pt is digitalized to reduce the ventricular rate and given IV Lasix for systolic heart failure.

2. TWO OR MORE INTER-RELATED CONDITIONS, EACH POTENTIALLY MEETING THE DEFINITION OF PRINCIPAL DIAGNOSIS

"When there are two or more interrelated conditions (such as diseases in the same ICD-10-CM chapter or manifestations characteristically associated with a certain disease) potentially meeting the definition of principal diagnosis, either condition may be sequenced first, unless the circumstances of the admission, the therapy provided, the Tabular List, or the Alphabetic Index indicate otherwise." (OCG II.B).

> **EXAMPLE** Patient is admitted with respiratory failure due to severe exacerbation of COPD. A pulmonary consultant is involved. Treatment includes IV antibiotics, steroids, oxygen, pulse oximetry, and aggressive respiratory therapy modalities. Either may be sequenced as principal diagnosis.

3. UNCERTAIN DIAGNOSIS

"If the diagnosis documented at the time of discharge is qualified as 'probable,' 'suspected,' 'likely,' 'questionable,' 'possible,' 'still to be ruled out,' 'compatible with,' 'consistent with,' or other similar terms indicating uncertainty, code the condition as if it existed or was established.

The bases for these guidelines are the diagnostic workup, arrangements for further workup or observation, and initial therapeutic approach that correspond most closely with the established diagnosis." (OCG Section II.H).

This guideline is applicable only to inpatient admissions, not outpatient visits.

Exception: Code only confirmed cases of HIV infection/illness, COVID-19, Zika, and influenza due to certain viruses, e.g., H1N1, avian, etc. (J09-J10).

Other terms that indicate **uncertainty** are "indicative of," "suggestive of," "comparable with," "appears to be," and "concern for."

> **EXAMPLE** "RLL pneumonia likely due to aspiration." Assign code J69.0 for aspiration pneumonia.

"Borderline" diagnoses documented at the time of discharge are also considered confirmed, unless ICD-10 has a specific code, e.g., borderline diabetes (R73.03).

"Rule out" conditions documented at discharge are ambiguous and should be clarified whether ruled-in or ruled-out. "Evidence of" is considered definitive, not uncertain.

The key issue for coding an uncertain diagnosis is to ensure the uncertain condition is not ruled out and is not stated otherwise at the time of discharge. At the time of discharge may mean in the final discharge note, when a consultant has signed off, or in the discharge summary.

If an uncertain diagnosis is determined to not be present, not clinically supported, or ruled out by the time of discharge, it would not be considered an uncertain diagnosis. For example, a code for "possible pneumonia" would not be assigned if antibiotics were discontinued before discharge or a full course of treatment.

4. CODES FOR SYMPTOMS, SIGNS, AND ILL-DEFINED CONDITIONS

"Codes for symptoms, signs, and ill-defined conditions from Chapter 18 are not to be used as principal diagnosis when a related definitive diagnosis has been established." (OCG Section II.A).

> **EXAMPLE** Syncope due to cardiac arrhythmia. Cardiac arrhythmia is the principal diagnosis; syncope is a secondary diagnosis.

Do not assign a separate code at all for signs and symptoms that are routinely associated with a disease process or when a related definitive diagnosis has been established (confirmed) as the cause. See OCG Sections I.B.4 and I.C.18.a and b.

> **EXAMPLE** Viral gastroenteritis with fever, abdominal pain, nausea and vomiting. Code only viral gastroenteritis.

When applying this rule, remember that Rule #3 treats uncertain diagnoses as "established."

EXAMPLE   Fever possibly due to UTI. Code UTI only.

See *Signs, Symptoms, and Unspecified Codes* for further details.

5. ORIGINAL TREATMENT PLAN NOT CARRIED OUT

"Sequence as the principal diagnosis the condition, which after study occasioned the admission to the hospital, even though treatment may not have been carried out due to unforeseen circumstances." (OCG Section II.F).

EXAMPLE   A patient with cholecystitis was admitted to the hospital for a cholecystectomy. Prior to surgery, the patient fell and sustained a left femur fracture. The surgery was canceled and a hip ORIF was performed on the second hospital day.

The principal diagnosis remains cholecystitis, since it necessitated the admission to the hospital. The fractured femur is sequenced as a secondary diagnosis since it occurred during the hospital stay.

6. COMPLICATIONS OF SURGERY AND OTHER MEDICAL CARE

"When the admission is for treatment of a complication resulting from surgery or other medical care, the complication code is sequenced as the principal diagnosis. If the complication is classified to the T80-T88 series and the code lacks the necessary specificity in describing the complication, an additional code for the specific complication should be assigned." (OCG Section II.G).

See *Complications of Care* section for further details.

EXAMPLES   Patient is readmitted with wound dehiscence two days following a hysterectomy. Sequence the wound dehiscence (T81.31Xa) as the principal diagnosis.

Patient is admitted with respiratory failure due to large iatrogenic pneumothorax three days following outpatient thoracentesis for malignant pleural effusion. Iatrogenic pneumothorax (J95.811) is the principal diagnosis.

7. ADMISSION FROM OBSERVATION UNITS

Admission from medical observation: "When a patient is admitted to an observation unit for a medical condition, which either worsens or does not improve, and is subsequently admitted as an inpatient of the same hospital for this same medical condition, the principal diagnosis would be the medical condition which led to the hospital admission." (OCG Section II.I.1).

Sometimes the reason for transition from observation is not entirely clear in the record and may require thoughtful interpretation of the clinical circumstances or even a query for clarification.

On occasion, a patient is treated as observation for several days before it's recognized that no inpatient order was given. The principal diagnosis must be something that still required management and was the focus of inpatient care at the time the inpatient order was written.

> **EXAMPLE** A patient is treated in an observation unit for 18 hours with dehydration, then admitted as an inpatient for low oxygen saturations and acute exacerbation of COPD. AECOPD is the principal diagnosis.

Admission from postoperative observation: "When a patient is admitted to an observation unit to monitor a condition (or complication) that develops following outpatient surgery, and then is subsequently admitted as an inpatient of the same hospital, hospitals should apply the Uniform Hospital Discharge Data Set (UHDDS) definition of principal diagnosis as "that condition established after study to be chiefly responsible for occasioning the admission of the patient to the hospital for care." (OCG Section II.I.2).

8. ADMISSION FROM OUTPATIENT SURGERY

"When a patient receives surgery in the hospital's outpatient surgery department and is subsequently admitted [directly] for continuing inpatient care at the same hospital, the following guidelines should be followed in selecting the principal diagnosis for the inpatient admission:

- If the reason for the inpatient admission is a complication, assign the complication as the principal diagnosis.
- If no complication, or other condition, is documented as the reason for the inpatient admission, assign the reason for the outpatient surgery as the principal diagnosis.
- If the reason for the inpatient admission is another condition unrelated to the surgery, assign the unrelated condition as the principal diagnosis." (OCG II.J). See also OCG II.I.2.

Note that the surgical procedure is also coded.

> **EXAMPLES** Patient admitted for postoperative bleeding following outpatient TURP; postoperative bleeding is the principal diagnosis.
>
> Patient being observed for 24 hours following lumbar laminectomy develops rapid atrial fibrillation requiring admission; atrial fibrillation would be the principal diagnosis.
>
> Elderly patient with chronic cholecystitis admitted for 3 days following uncomplicated elective lap cholecystectomy without further explanation before being transferred to a SNF; chronic cholecystitis is the principal diagnosis.

9. TWO OR MORE COMPARATIVE/CONTRASTING DIAGNOSES

"In those rare instances when two or more contrasting or comparative diagnoses are documented as "either/or" (or similar terminology), they are sequenced according to the circumstances of the admission. If no further determination can be made as to which diagnosis should be principal, either diagnosis may be sequenced first." (OCG Section II.D).

> **EXAMPLE** "Acute pancreatitis vs. acute cholecystitis." Depending on the circumstances of admission, either may be sequenced as principal diagnosis.

Other (secondary) diagnoses are defined as "all conditions that coexist at the time of admission, that develop subsequently, or that affect the treatment received and/or the length of stay. Diagnoses that relate to an earlier episode which have no bearing on the current hospital stay are to be excluded." (OCG Section III).

The **definition** for "other diagnoses" is "interpreted as additional conditions [either present on admission or occurring during admission] that affect patient care in terms of requiring:

- Clinical evaluation, or
- Therapeutic treatment, or
- Diagnostic procedures, or
- Extended length of hospital stay, or
- Increased nursing care and/or monitoring."

Conditions which are documented but do not meet one of these five requirements should not be reported. As with all codes, clinical evidence should be present in the medical record to support code assignment.

Chronic conditions such as hypertension, congestive heart failure, asthma, COPD, Parkinson's disease, diabetes mellitus, and many others typically require chronic treatment and meet the above definition.

Coding Clinics 2008 Third Quarter p. 12, and 2013 Second Quarter, p. 33, state that the terms exacerbated and decompensated indicate "there has been a flare-up (acute phase) of a chronic condition." Therefore a chronic condition described as **decompensated** or **exacerbated** may be coded as "acute."

Obesity and morbid obesity are always considered clinically significant when documented (Coding Clinic 2011 Third Quarter). However, documentation of "CHF" on an anesthesia assessment, without any further indications of ongoing treatment, does not suggest clinical significance and thus the condition would not be reported.

The **Uncertain Diagnosis** rule also applies to the assignment of secondary diagnoses (OCG Section III).

Abnormal findings. Laboratory, x-ray, pathology, and other diagnostic results are not coded and reported unless the provider indicates their clinical significance. If the findings are outside the normal range and the attending provider has ordered other tests to evaluate the condition or prescribed treatment, it is appropriate to ask the provider whether the abnormal finding should be added (OCG Section III.B).

> **EXAMPLES** Patient with serum sodium of 125. Do not code unless physician states "hyponatremia."
> Small cell carcinoma on pathology report must be documented by a provider in the body of the medical record.

Greater specificity. Although perhaps not widely understood, it has been an acceptable inpatient coding practice to assign greater specificity of established diagnoses based on diagnostic studies that have been interpreted by a physician.

According to Coding Clinic 2013 First Quarter, p. 28, "If the x-ray report provides additional information regarding the site for a condition that the provider has already diagnosed, it would be appropriate to assign a code to identify the specificity that is documented in the x-ray report."

The same can be said for other situations where ICD-10 provides greater specificity for an established diagnosis such as:

- Laterality and involved artery for a diagnosed nonspecific CVA from CT or MRI/MRA
- Location or involved artery for an unspecified diagnosis of STEMI obtained from the EKG

A good compliance "rule of thumb" is to never assign greater specificity from an interpreted diagnostic test result without provider documentation if it will impact the DRG resulting in higher payment.

> **EXAMPLE** Documented heart failure with echocardiogram report showing "diastolic dysfunction." Do not assign diastolic heart failure; instead query the provider.

Conditions from prior encounters. "Documentation from the current encounter should clearly reflect those diagnoses that are current and relevant for that encounter…When reporting recurring conditions and the recurring condition is still valid for the outpatient encounter or inpatient admission, the recurring condition should be documented in the medical record with each encounter/admission… It is inappropriate to go back to previous encounter(s) to retrieve a diagnosis without physician confirmation." (Coding Clinic 2013 Third Quarter p. 27).

Therefore, it would be appropriate to query the physician regarding a condition from a previous encounter based on indicators from the current encounter and pertinent information from the previous encounter if the condition meets the definition of a secondary diagnosis (being treated, clinically evaluated, etc.).

According to OCG Section III, "Diagnoses that relate to an earlier episode which have **no bearing on the current hospital stay** are to be excluded. Some providers include… resolved conditions or diagnoses… from a previous admission that have no bearing on the current stay. Such conditions are not to be reported and are coded only if required by hospital policy."

The 2019 AHIMA/ACDIS compliant query practice brief also states: "Prior encounter information may be referenced in queries for clinical clarification and/or validation if it is clinically pertinent to the present encounter. However, it is inappropriate to 'mine' a previous encounter's documentation to generate queries not related to the current encounter." Therefore, a diagnosis from a previous encounter that **does have a bearing** on the current stay should be documented, so it can be currently coded.

For example, the OCG requires that if AIDS or HIV disease has ever been previously diagnosed, code B20 must be assigned on every subsequent encounter. If not documented on the current episode of care with a confirmed diagnosis of AIDS or HIV disease in prior records, a query is the proper method for obtaining this information.

OVERVIEW AND GUIDELINES

In general, coding rules for children (older than 28 days) are the same as adults. Perinatal and neonatal (≤ 28 days) have some unique rules.

Principal diagnosis for newborn record. When coding the birth episode in a newborn record, the principal diagnosis is assigned a code from category Z38, Liveborn infants according to place of birth and type of delivery. For example:

- Z3800 Single liveborn infant, delivered vaginally in hospital
- Z3831 Twin liveborn infant, delivered by cesarean in hospital

A category code Z38 is assigned only once to a newborn at the time of birth. If a newborn was transferred from another institution, a code from category Z38 would not be used at the receiving hospital.

Present on admission. Newborns are not considered admitted until after birth. Therefore, any condition present at birth or that developed in utero is considered present on admission. POA criteria for children are the same as adults.

Perinatal period. For coding and reporting purposes the perinatal period is defined as before birth through the 28th day following birth. Perinatal conditions are included in Chapter 16: "Certain conditions originating in the perinatal period" categories P00-P96. These codes are never used in the maternal record.

Perinatal conditions. All clinically significant conditions noted on the newborn examination should be coded (OCG I.16.a.6). A condition is clinically significant if it requires:

- clinical evaluation, or
- therapeutic treatment, or
- diagnostic procedures, or
- extended length of hospital stay, or
- increased nursing care and/or monitoring, or
- ***has implications for future healthcare needs.***

The above guidelines are the same as the general coding guidelines for additional diagnoses, except "has implications for future healthcare needs" (e.g., murmur that needs further evaluation, or sacral dimple requiring follow-up US or MRI).

Should a condition originate in the perinatal period and continue throughout the life of the patient, the perinatal code should continue to be used regardless of the patient's age (OCG I.C.16.a.4), e.g., pulmonary hypertension of newborn (P29.30).

If a newborn has a condition that may be either due to the birth process or community acquired and the documentation does not indicate which it is, the default is due to the birth process and a P00-P96 code should be used. If the condition is community-acquired, these codes should not be assigned (OCG I.C.16.a.5). A provider query may be necessary.

Preterm infants. Defined as birth prior to the beginning of the 37th week. Preterm and premature are considered synonymous terms. Providers sometimes utilize different criteria in determining prematurity. A code for prematurity should not be assigned unless it is documented.

For accurate APR-DRG assignment of preterm infants, assign the appropriate code from categories P05 (Newborn disorders related to slow fetal growth and fetal malnutrition) and P07 (Newborn disorders related to short gestation and low birth weight) based on the recorded birth weight and estimated gestational age.

When both birth weight and gestational age are available, assign two codes from category P07 with the code for birth weight sequenced before the code for gestational age (OCG I.C.16.d). Example:

- P07.02 Extremely low birth weight newborn, 500-749 grams
- P07.31 Preterm infant, gestational age 28 completed weeks

Codes from P07 can continue to be used for a child or an adult who was premature or had a low birth weight as a newborn which continues to affect the patient's current status (OCG I.C.16.e).

Congenital disorders. When a malformation/deformation or chromosomal abnormality is documented, assign an appropriate code(s) from code categories Q00-Q99, Congenital malformations, deformations, and chromosomal abnormalities. For example, atrial septal defect (Q21.1) and isomerism of atrial appendages (Q20.6).

When a malformation/deformation or chromosomal abnormality does not have a unique code assignment, assign additional code(s) for any manifestations that may be present. For example, heterotaxy syndrome may include intestinal malrotation, biliary atresia, atrial isomerism, and other types of congenital heart disease. Because there is not a unique code for heterotaxy syndrome, all the different manifestations would be coded separately.

When the code assignment specifically identifies the malformation/deformation or chromosomal abnormality, manifestations that are an inherent component of the anomaly are not coded separately. Additional codes should be assigned for manifestations that are not an inherent component.

Q00-Q99 codes may be used throughout the life of the patient. If a congenital malformation/deformity has been corrected, a personal history code should be used to identify the history of the malformation or deformity. Although present at birth, a malformation/deformation or chromosomal abnormality may not be identified until later in life.

Child abuse. If the documentation in the medical record states abuse or neglect, it is coded as confirmed (T74.-). It is coded as suspected if it is documented as suspected (T76.-). The code from categories T74.- or T76.- are *sequenced first* followed by any accompanying injury or mental health code(s) due to the abuse.

References

- Official Coding Guidelines I.C. 16 and 17 and I.C.19.f
- UpToDate.com: Late preterm infants
- Coding Clinics: 2018 Q2 p. 6; 2017 Q4 p. 20-22; 2017 Q2 p. 7; 2017 Q1 p. 29-30; 2016 Q4 p. 54-55.

OVERVIEW

All ICD-10-PCS procedure codes are alphanumeric 7-digit codes. The most challenging part of constructing and assigning a PCS code is determining the specific root operation (3rd digit) and the approach (5th digit), both of which can impact DRG assignment. The 7th digit qualifier specifying the procedure as "diagnostic" rather than "therapeutic" is important particularly for excisional biopsies.

ICD-10-PCS includes standard operative terms in the alphabetical index, such as cholecystectomy, which is then translated to the appropriate root operation, but does not include eponyms (e.g., Whipple procedure). The physician is not expected to use the specific root operation terms in the · PCS code description. It is the coder's responsibility to determine which PCS definitions fit the medical record documentation.

For example, the main term Cholecystectomy refers to Excision, Gallbladder (0FB4) or Resection, Gallbladder (0FT4). The definitions of these two root operations (excision and resection) will determine which one to select.

Root Operations. To help distinguish the different root operations, we have divided them into six groups that share similar characteristics:

1. Remove a body part
2. Implant or move a body part
3. Remove matter from a body part
4. Procedures on a tubular body part
5. Procedures with a device
6. Other procedures

These different groups include the root operations, their definitions and site, and examples of PCS procedure codes for some of more commonly performed surgical procedures to help guide you in procedural code selection.

Approach. The seven techniques, or the "**approach**," to reach the procedural site are:

- **External**: directly on skin or by applying external force through the skin or membrane (closed reduction of a fracture, skin lesion biopsy, tonsillectomy)
- Through the skin or mucous membrane:
  - **Open**: cutting through the skin or mucous membrane (abdominal hysterectomy, colon resection, CABG)
  - **Percutaneous**: puncture/minor incision to reach the operative site (paracentesis, insertion of pacemaker lead, needle biopsy of liver)
  - **Percutaneous endoscopic**: percutaneous with visualization by endoscope (knee arthroscopy, lap cholecystectomy)
- Through a natural or artificial opening (urethra, esophagus, colostomy)
  - **Via natural or artificial opening** (vaginal endometrial ablation, ET intubation)
  - **Via natural or artificial opening with endoscopy:** with visualization by endoscope (bronchoscopy)
  - **Via natural or artificial opening with percutaneous endoscopy:** entry through a natural/artificial opening but with percutaneous endoscopy to aid in performing the procedure (EGD with gastric biopsy, lap-assisted vaginal hysterectomy)

Diagnostic Qualifier. The 7th digit qualifier "X" (diagnostic) is used to identify excision, extraction and drainage procedures that are exclusively diagnostic procedures, i.e., biopsies. If there is a therapeutic component to the procedure the qualifier Z (no qualifier) should be used.

An "excisional biopsy" of an entire mass or lesion if completely excised would be therapeutic as well as diagnostic, and coded with a 7th digit of Z, not X "diagnostic" for biopsy. For example, "excisional biopsy" of left thigh abscess that was completely excised is coded 0JBM0ZZ and considered an OR procedure.

REMOVE A BODY PART

RESECTION	Cutting out or off, without replacement	All of a body part

- **Cholecystectomy**: *0FT40ZZ Resection of Gallbladder, Open; Laparoscopic: 0FT44ZZ Resection of Gallbladder, Perc. Endoscopic*
- **Lung lobectomy**: *0BTC0ZZ Resection of Right Upper Lung Lobe, Open*
- **Sigmoidectomy**: *0DTN0ZZ Resection of Sigmoid Colon, Open*
- **Thoracoscopic lobectomy of lung**: *0BTC4ZZ Resection of Right Upper Lung Lobe, Percutaneous Endoscopic*

EXCISION	Cutting out or off, without replacement	Portion of a body part

- **Excisional wound debridement, leg**: *0JBN0ZZ Excision of Right Lower Leg Subcutaneous Tissue and Fascia, Open*
- **Liver biopsy**: *0FB03ZX Excision of liver, Percutaneous, Diagnostic*
- **Lumbar laminectomy**: *0SB00ZZ Excision of Lumbar Vertebral Joint, Open*
- **Pelvic bone biopsy**: *0QB30ZX Excision of Left Pelvic Bone, Open, Diagnostic*
- **Partial lobectomy**: *0BBL4ZZ Excision of Left Lung, Perc. Endoscopic*
- **Transbronchial lung biopsy**: *0BBJ8ZX Excision of Left Lower Lung Lobe, Via Natural or Artificial Opening Endoscopic, Diagnostic*

DETACHMENT	Cutting off without replacement	All or a portion: Upper or lower extremities

- **BKA**: *0Y6J0Z1 Detachment at Left Lower Leg, High, Open*
- **AKA**: *0Y6C0Z3 Detachment at Right Upper Leg, Low, Open*
- **Amputation of toe**: *0Y6Y0Z2 Detachment at Left 5th Toe, Mid, Open*

DESTRUCTION	Physical eradication	All or a portion of a body part

- **Cardiac ablation**: *02563ZZ Destruction of Right Atrium, Percutaneous*
- **Sigmoidoscopy with rectal polyp fulguration**: *0D5P8ZZ Destruction of Rectum, via Natural or Artificial Opening, Endoscopic*

EXTRACTION	Pulling or stripping out or off	All or a portion of a body part

- **D&C**: *0UDB7ZZ Extraction of Endometrium, Via Natural or Artificial Opening*
- **Non-excisional debridement rt upper leg**: *0JDL0ZZ Extraction of Right Upper Leg Subcutaneous Tissue and Fascia, Open*

IMPLANT OR MOVE A BODY PART

TRANSPLANTATION	Putting in a living body part taken from a person or animal	All or some of a body part

- **Kidney transplant:** *0TY10Z0 Transplantation of Left Kidney, Allogeneic, Open*

REATTACHMENT	Putting back a separated body part to its normal location	All or some of a body part

- **Reattachment of rt index finger**: *0XMP0ZZ Reattachment of Left Index Finger, Open*

REPOSITION	Moving a body part to its normal location or other suitable location	All or portion of a body part

- **ORIF Femur**: *0QSB04Z Reposition Right Lower Femur with Internal Fixation Device, Open*
- **Closed reduction of dislocated shoulder joint**: *0RSJXZZ Reposition Rt Shoulder Joint, External*

TRANSFER	Moving a body part to function for a similar body part	All or a portion of a body part

- **Tendon transfer:** *0LXM0ZZ Transfer Left Upper Leg Tendon, Open*
- **Colon interposition following esophageal resection:** *0DXE0Z5 Transfer Large Intestine to Esophagus, Open*

REMOVE MATTER FROM A BODY PART

DRAINAGE	Taking or letting out fluids and/gases	Within a body part

- **Abdominal paracentesis:** *0W9G3ZZ Drainage of Peritoneal Cavity, Percutaneous*
- **I&D of perianal abscess**: *0D9QXZZ Drainage of Anus, External*
- **Drainage of retropharyngeal abscess:** *0W960ZZ Drainage of Neck, Open*

EXTIRPATION	Taking or cutting out solid matter	Within a body part

- **Carotid endarterectomy:** *03CH4ZZ Extirpation of Matter from Right Common Carotid Artery, Percutaneous Endoscopic*

FRAGMENTATION	Breaking solid matter into pieces	Within a body part

- **ESWL kidney:** *0TF4XZZ Fragmentation in Left Kidney Pelvis, External*

PROCEDURES ON A TUBULAR BODY PART

DILATION	Expanding an orifice or the lumen of a tubular body part	Tubular body part

- **PTCA with stent:** *027034Z Dilation of Coronary Artery, One Artery with Drug-eluting Intraluminal Device, Percutaneous*

RESTRICTION	Partially closing an orifice or the lumen of a tubular body part	Tubular body part

- **Gastroesophageal fundoplication:** *0DV48ZZ Restriction of Esophagogastric Junction, Via Natural or Artificial Opening Endoscopic*

OCCLUSION	Completely closing an orifice or the lumen	Tubular body part

- **Ligation of bleeding gastric artery:** *04L20ZZ Occlusion of Gastric Artery, Open Approach*

BYPASS	Altering route of passage of the contents	Tubular body part

- **CABG:** *02100AW Bypass Coronary Artery, One Artery from Aorta with Autologous Arterial Tissue, Open Approach*
- **Dialysis AV Shunt:** *031C0ZF Bypass Left Radial Artery to Lower Arm Vein, Open*
- **Tracheostomy:** *0B110F4 Bypass Trachea to Cutaneous with Tracheostomy Device, Open*

PROCEDURES WITH A DEVICE

REPLACEMENT	Putting in a device that replaces a body part	Some of all of a body part

- **Total hip replacement:** *0SR90JZ Replacement of Right Hip Joint with Synthetic Substitute, Open*
- **Total knee replacement***: 0SRD0J9 Replacement of Left Knee Joint with Synthetic Substitute, Cemented, Open*
- **Aortic valve replacement:** *02RF0KZ Replacement of Aortic Valve with Nonautologous Tissue Substitute, Open*
- **TAVR***: 02RF4JZ Replacement of Aortic Valve with Synthetic Substitute, Percutaneous Endoscopic*

INSERTION	Putting in a nonbiological device that monitors, assists, performs, or prevents a physiological function	In or on a body part

- **Cardiac pacemaker:** *0JH636Z Insertion of Pacemaker, Dual Chamber into Chest Subcutaneous Tissue and Fascia, Percutaneous*
- **Defibrillator***: 0JH609Z Insertion of Cardiac Resynchronization Defibrillator Pulse Generator into Chest Subcutaneous Tissue and Fascia, Open*

REMOVAL	Taking out or off a device	In or on a body part

- **Cardiac pacemaker generator removal:** *0JPT0PZ Removal of Cardiac Rhythm Related Device from Trunk Subcutaneous Tissue and Fascia, Open*
- **PEG tube removal:** *0DP6XUZ Removal of Feeding Device from Stomach, via Natural or Artificial Opening, Endoscopic*

REVISION	Correcting a malfunctioning or displaced device	In or on a body part

- **Adjustment of position of pacemaker lead:** *02WA3MZ Revision of Cardiac Lead in Heart, Percutaneous*
- **Revision of rt hip arthroplasty***: 0SW90JZ Revision of Synthetic Substitute in Right Hip Joint, Open*

SUPPLEMENT	Putting in a device that physically reinforces and/or augments the function of a body part	In or on a body part

- **Incisional hernia repair with mesh:** *0WUF0JZ Supplement Abdominal Wall with Synthetic Substitute, Open*
- **New acetabular liner in a previous hip replacement:** *0QU50JZ Supplement Left Acetabulum with Synthetic Substitute, Open*

CHANGE	Taking out or off a device from a body part without cutting or puncturing the skin or a mucous membrane.	In or on a body part

- **Urinary catheter change:** *0T2DX0Z Change Drainage Device in Urethra, External*

OTHER PROCEDURES

FUSION	Joining together portions of an articular body part and rendering it immobile	Joint

- **Cervical spinal fusion:** *0RG2371 Fusion of Two or More Cervical Vertebral Joints with Autologous Tissue Substitute, Posterior approach, Posterior column, Percutaneous*
- **Arthroscopic rt subtalar arthrodesis with internal fixation:** *0SGH44Z Fusion of Rt Tarsal Joint with Internal Fixation Device, Perc. Endoscopic*
- **Posterior lumbar fusion:** *0SG007J Fusion Lumbar Joint w Autologous Tissue Substitute, Posterior Approach, Anterior Column, Open*

CONTROL	Stopping, or attempting to stop, postprocedural or other acute bleeding	General anatomical region

- **Control of postoperative GI bleeding:** *0W3P8ZZ Control Bleeding in Gastrointestinal Tract, Via Natural or Artificial Opening Endoscopic*
- **Cauterization of a bleeding cerebral artery:** *0W310ZZ Control Bleeding in Cranial Cavity, Open*

INSPECTION	Visual and/or manual exploration	All of some of a body part

- **Exploratory laparotomy:** *0WJG0ZZ Inspection of Peritoneal Cavity, Open*

RELEASE	Freeing body part from constraint by cutting or by use of force	Around a body part

- **Peritoneal adhesiolysis**: *0DNW3ZZ Release Peritoneum, Percutaneous*

REPAIR	Restoring, to the extent possible, a body part to its normal anatomic structure and function	All of some of a body part

- **Colostomy takedown:** *0DQE0ZZ Repair Large Intestine, Open*
- **Suture of facial laceration:** *0HQ1XZZ Repair Face Skin, External*

DIVISION	Cutting into/separating or transecting	Within a body part

- **Neurotomy:** *018F0ZZ Division of Sciatic Nerve, Open Approach*
- **Spinal cordotomy:** *008X3ZZ Division of Thoracic Spinal Cord, Percutaneous*

*Note: Two root operations not included above are "**Creation**" which is for gender reassignment surgery and "**Alteration**" which are procedures for cosmetic purposes.*

Other Non-OR procedure examples that impact certain MS-DRGs:

- **Cardiac Catheterization (DRGs 216-218, 222-225, 233-234, 286-287):** *4A023N7 Measurement of Cardiac Sampling and Pressure, Left Heart, Percutaneous Approach*
- **Mechanical Ventilation (DRGs 207-208, 870):** *5A1935Z: Respiratory ventilation < 24 consecutive hours; 5A1945Z: 24-96 hours; 5A1955Z: > 96 hours.*
- **Rehab Therapy (DRG 895):** *HZ31ZZZ Individual Counseling for Substance Abuse Treatment, Behavioral*
- **TPA (DRG 61-63):** *3E03317 Introduction of Other Thrombolytic into Peripheral Vein, Percutaneous*

Medicare MS-DRGs are used primarily for patients over age 65. To better accommodate the entire patient population, both adult and pediatric, 3M and the National Association of Children's Hospitals and Related Institutions collaboratively developed the 3M APR-DRG system in 1990.

APR-DRGs are a proprietary, severity-adjusted system used to adjust inpatient claims data for severity of illness and risk of mortality. More than 30 states have adopted APR-DRGs for inpatient payment or quality reporting for either Medicaid or Blue Cross.

APR-DRGs are similar in structure to MS-DRGs, with generally comparable base DRGs split into severity subclasses based on secondary diagnoses. Each APR base DRG has four subclasses of severity of illness (SOI) and four subclasses of risk of mortality (ROM), as opposed to as many as three severity levels for MS-DRGs using MCCs and CCs. See Table 1 below. Consequently, there are almost twice as many APR-DRGs than MS-DRGs.

Table 1: **MS-DRG VS. APR-DRG**

MS-DRG	APR-DRG
Main Driver:	Main Driver:
Principal Diagnosis or Surgical Procedure	Principal Diagnosis or Surgical Procedure
Secondary Diagnosis:	Secondary Diagnosis:
MCC	SOI 4 (Extreme)
CC	SOI 3 (Major)
Non-CC	SOI 2 (Moderate)
	SOI 1 (Minor)

APR-DRG assignment. Assignment of APR-DRGs is highly complex; statistical algorithms and rerouting logic are used to determine the final DRG and severity subclass. By comparison, MS-DRGs are straightforward, intuitive, and transparent.

The APR-DRG system assigns discharges to a DRG SOI subclass as follows:

1. Assign base DRG by principal diagnosis and principal procedure.
2. Determine the standard SOI level for each secondary diagnosis.
3. Assign the final DRG/SOI subclass based on the combination and hierarchy of all diagnoses.

Table 2: **APR-DRG 139**

Base DRG	SOI	DRG Description	V38.0 Weight*
139	1	Other Pneumonia	0.4890
139	2	Other Pneumonia	0.6407
139	3	Other Pneumonia	0.9409
139	4	Other Pneumonia	1.7976

Weights are for Ohio Medicaid. Weights vary by state and payer.

The more common MS-DRG MCCs are classified in APR-DRG as SOI Level 3 or 4, CCs are typically SOI 2, and most non-CCs are SOI 1. A few non-CCs are assigned SOI 2.

While a single MCC or CC determines the MS-DRG, multiple secondary diagnoses can influence the APR-DRG. However, not all secondary diagnoses make a difference in the final APR-DRG assignment. In most circumstances, only two or three secondary diagnoses with the highest SOI levels are needed to determine the final APR-DRG SOI subclass.

Table 3: **APR-DRG SOI Levels**

Combination of Secondary Diagnosis SOI Levels	APR-DRG SOI Subclass*
Two SOI 4, or One SOI 4 and two SOI 3	4 (Extreme)
Two SOI 3, or One SOI 3 and two SOI 2	3 (Major)
One or more SOI 2	2 (Moderate)

APR rerouting logic, exclusions, and patient age may result in a different SOI subclass.

The standard SOI level is included in the *Comorbid Conditions* section of this guide although APR logic may result in a different SOI subclass.

A **risk of mortality (ROM)** score with four levels is also assigned to each APR-DRG based on principal and secondary diagnoses as with SOI. ROM may impact certain mortality reporting metrics.

Optimal APR-DRG severity of illness. CDI should assign and group inpatient cases using the APR-DRG grouper when it is available for APR-DRG payers, such as Medicaid. Likewise, the MS-DRG grouper should be used for Medicare and other MS-DRG payers.

If the APR-DRG grouper is not available, obtaining documentation of a combination of two or three MCC/CCs will usually approximate the expected APR-DRG SOI (see Table 4). While imperfect, the result will usually be a solid SOI classification without an APR-DRG grouper.

Documentation and coding of at least **two MCCs and/or CCs** also guards against payer DRG changes, since audit contractors often focus on cases with only one MCC or CC.

Table 4: **Severity Impact Using MCC/CCs**

Strategy	Description
Two MCCs	If only one MCC is identified and clinical indicators of another MCC are present, query the physician for this second MCC.
One MCC + Two CCs	If only one MCC is identified and there are no clinical indicators for a second MCC, search and query for up to two additional CCs.
Two CCs	If there are no clinical indicators for any MCC, search and query for up to two CCs.

The ICD-10 coding convention **"etiology/manifestation" (E/M)** requires the underlying condition (cause/etiology) to be sequenced first followed by its manifestation (effect). It applies only to a very *limited* number of conditions and their manifestations that are specifically identified by ICD-10 Index entries and Tabular instructional notes. See OCG I.A.13.

Wherever such a combination exists, there is a **"code first"** note at the manifestation code and/or **"use additional code"** note at the etiology code. These instructional notes indicate the proper sequencing order of the codes, etiology followed by manifestation.

In some cases the manifestation code includes **"in diseases classified elsewhere"** in the code title. Codes with this title are a component of the E/M convention. They cannot be used as a principal diagnosis or first-listed code.

> EXAMPLES Malignant pleural effusion - "Code first underlying neoplasm"
> Pyelonephritis due to multiple myeloma - "Code first underlying disease"
> Bleeding esophageal varices in liver cirrhosis - "Code first underlying disease"
> Type II MI due to anemia- "Code first the underlying cause"

E/M convention does not apply to other conditions. Conditions and codes outside of the E/M convention are not subject to this rule. Sequencing of all other diagnoses is based on the circumstances of admission and the definition of principal diagnosis, unless there is other authoritative coding direction. Any such condition documented as "due to" or that happens to be a manifestation or etiology of another plays no role in sequencing.

> EXAMPLES "Encephalopathy due to UTI" or "Acute renal failure due to dehydration" does not require sequencing the etiology (UTI or dehydration) as the principal diagnosis.

Signs and symptoms of an established diagnosis are never sequenced first. Signs and symptoms routinely associated with an established condition are not separately coded at all.

The purpose of clinical documentation is to accurately capture a patient's medical condition. Documentation not only guides patient care but it also forms the basis for hospital statistics and, most importantly for the purposes of this guide, for proper code assignment. If clinical documentation were easy, however, we wouldn't need CDI programs.

One of the fundamental challenges for physicians is keeping abreast not only with updates to clinical criteria for numerous conditions but also with specific terminology to ensure proper code assignment. Of course, sometimes solutions bring their own problems: some clinicians have become overzealous in documenting conditions that are commonly queried. This is in part because they're trying to be good team players, but in some cases it's also to avoid queries which some find annoying and take up precious time. As a result, some hospitals are plagued with clinically invalid "over-diagnoses" that lead to improper DRG reimbursement and payer denials.

Here's the difficulty in a nutshell:

If your clinical documentation doesn't support the diagnoses, the hospital will lose revenue. If the clinical documentation results in claims that are not valid, the hospital could face serious penalties for claims that result in over-payment.

Roots of confusion: OCG vs. CMS

The Official Guidelines for Coding and Reporting (OCG) Section I.A.19 in 2016 stated: *"The assignment of a diagnosis code is based on the provider's diagnostic statement that the condition exists. The provider's statement that the patient has a particular condition is sufficient. Code assignment is not based on clinical criteria used by the provider to establish the diagnosis."*

You'd be forgiven for wondering if this OCG guideline means that clinical validation of documented conditions is no longer required for code assignment on claims. In response, Coding Clinic 2016 Fourth Quarter p. 147, tried to clarify:

"Coders should not be disregarding physician documentation and deciding on their own, based on clinical criteria, abnormal test results, etc., whether or not a condition should be coded."

Which may leave many wondering that CDI and clinical validation are no longer required.

The answer is unequivocal: **clinical validation is an absolute statutory and regulatory imperative** for claims submission.

The latest guidance for clinical validation is AHIMA's "Clinical Validation: The Next Level" (January 2019) practice brief, which states that clinical validation is

"the process of validating each diagnosis or procedure documented within the health record, ensuring it is supported by clinical evidence."

Moreover, AHIMA's Code of Ethics Principal 4.8 prohibits participating in, condoning, or being associated with dishonesty, fraud, abuse, or deception including "allowing patterns of optimizing or minimizing documentation and/or coding to impact payment..." and "coding when documentation does not justify the diagnoses or procedures that have been billed….."

The implications for clinical validation are clear from the statutes and regulations for billing and reimbursement:

- CMS RAC Statement of Work: "Clinical validation involves a clinical review of the case to see whether or not the patient truly possesses the conditions that were documented in the medical record."

- CMS Medicare Program Integrity Manual: "The purpose of DRG validation is to ensure that diagnostic and procedural information…coded and reported by the hospital on its claims matches the attending physician's description and the information contained in the medical record."

- The False Claims Act of 1863 imposes civil liability on any person (or organizations) who knowingly submits, or causes the submission of, a false or fraudulent claim to the Federal government.

The consequences of submitting clinically invalid diagnoses are numerous and can be severe: improper DRG reimbursement, excessive denials, unnecessary appeals, risk of regulatory audits and penalties. Over-coding leads to MCC/CC classification downgrades, as have occurred with AKI and encephalopathy. To add insult to injury, denials and appeals mostly serve to enrich audit contractors at the expense of the Medicare trust fund.

How to avoid inadequate documentation and false claims

Rely on authoritative sources. In this Guide we rely on authoritative, evidenced-based consensus criteria and guidelines for clinical validation. When you need more information, consult these excellent authoritative resources for some of the most commonly queried conditions, such as KDIGO for acute kidney injury, Sepsis-2 and Sepsis-3 consensus definitions for sepsis, and ASPEN or GLIM for malnutrition.

Make helpful clinical validation queries. To address those situations in which a physician documents a diagnosis which does not appear to be supported by the chart, the 2019 practice brief recommends a "clinical validation" query to the clinician requesting that the practitioner "confirm the presence of the condition and provide additional rationale." It is helpful if the person making the query can point to official consensus criteria to ensure that the basis of the query is clear.

When a clinician does not respond or responds to a query by confirming the diagnosis without providing further supporting information, the need for clinical evidence remains unmet and the diagnosis should not be reported on the claim.

Notice patterns. If there is a pattern of recurrent, clinically invalid diagnoses, a peer-to-peer intervention with a physician advisor can be helpful if your facility has one.

A hospital policy and procedure should be developed by a multi-disciplinary group of stakeholders, including CDI, coding, compliance, and the medical staff to address these high-risk diagnoses and ensure that invalid diagnoses are not reported on claims. When obviously invalid, the CDI team is certainly qualified to make a decision to omit a code, perhaps engaging a physician advisor for advice. After all, there are no consequences for removing a clinically invalid diagnosis code but more serious problems if you don't.

References

- CMS MLN Matters SE1121
- Clinical Validation: The Next Level of CDI. Journal of AHIMA (January 2019)
- CMS RAC Statement of Work 2014. Task 2.G.1.a.iii
- Cornell University Law School. Legal Information Institute: 31 U.S. Code § 3729—False claims
- Coding Clinic 2016 Fourth Quarter p. 147: Clinical Criteria and Code Assignment
- Coding Clinic 2017 Fourth Quarter p. 110: Omitting ICD-10-CM Codes.

Coding describes the process used to transform disease, injury, and procedure descriptions into alpha-numeric codes. The aggregation of clinical data into reportable categories supports requirements ranging from reimbursement to statistical analysis of diseases and therapeutic actions to public health surveillance.

Uniform Hospital Discharge Data Set (UHDDS). The UHDDS definitions are used by acute care hospitals to report codes and other inpatient data elements on the hospital claim in a consistent manner.

All diagnoses and significant procedures that affect the current hospital stay are to be reported on the claim. The claim form will permit up to 25 diagnoses, including the admitting diagnosis, and up to 25 procedure codes to be reported and submitted on the claim.

Inpatient Prospective Payment System (IPPS). In 1983 the IPPS system was introduced by the federal agency now known as the Centers for Medicare & Medicaid Services (CMS) as a means to curb skyrocketing healthcare costs for Medicare patients. The IPPS was designed to change hospital behavior through financial incentives that encourage more cost-efficient management of medical care.

Under the IPPS, the codes assigned to documented diagnoses and procedures in patient medical records also assign each patient to one of 765 categories, known as "Diagnosis Related Groups" (DRGs).

Diagnosis Related Groups (DRGs). DRG systems are inpatient classification schemes that categorize patients who share similar clinical characteristics and costs. Each inpatient discharge is assigned a DRG based on the ICD-10 codes on the hospital billing claim. Medicare adopted DRGs as a payment system in 1983 which were updated to MS-DRGs (Medicare Severity) in 2008. Another DRG system developed by 3M, APR-DRGs (All Patient Refined), is used as a payment methodology by many state Medicaid programs.

Each year, every DRG is assigned a fixed value (called "relative weight") applicable to all hospitals and used in calculating the reimbursement for all services provided during an inpatient admission.

A hospital-specific reimbursement rate is assigned to each hospital based on its costs associated with its particular patient population. For Medicare, this is known as the hospital's blended rate composed of a base rate plus add-ons for local wage variations, teaching hospitals, and hospitals with a disproportionate share of indigent patients.

The DRG payment is calculated by multiplying the relative weight for the DRG by the hospital's reimbursement rate. For example:

MS-DRG 293—Heart Failure	
Relative Weight (RW)	0.5899
Hospital Blended Rate	$6,000
MS-DRG Payment	$3,539
Geometric Length of Stay (GMLOS)	2.2

Relative weight is indicative of length of stay, severity of illness, resource utilization, and cost. Higher relative weight suggests a "sicker," more resource intensive patient.

GMLOS (geometric mean length of stay) is the national mean length of stay for a particular MS-DRG. By excluding outlier cases, the GMLOS reduces the effect of very high or low values, which would bias the mean if a simple average (arithmetic mean) is used.

The GMLOS is used to determine the per diem payment rate for patients transferred to a post-acute care setting for specified MS-DRGs. For example, if a patient is transferred to another acute care hospital before the GMLOS is reached, the hospital is paid twice the per diem rate for the first day of the stay, and the per diem rate for each subsequent day up to the full MS-DRG amount.

Case mix index (CMI). A hospital's CMI is the average of all DRG weights for a specific patient volume and time period. The CMI is proportional to reimbursement and the overall severity of illness of a patient population. A low CMI may indicate DRG assignments that do not adequately reflect the severity of illness, the resources used to treat patients, or the quality of care provided.

CMI calculation example:

Population: Medicare Inpatient Acute Care Time Period: 10/1/2021 to 9/30/2022				
DRG	DRG Description	Weight	# DCs	Total Wt.
291	CHF w MCC	1.2683	243	308.20
378	GI Hemorrhage w CC	0.9935	193	191.75
470	Major Joint Replacement	1.9003	286	543.49
871	Sepsis w MCC	1.8722	180	337.00
Sum			902	1380.44
CMI (Total Wt./# DCs)				1.5304
Reimbursement (# DCs × CMI) × Blended Rate ($6,000)				$8,282,525

MS-DRG assignment. MS-DRG assignment is driven by the principal diagnosis, secondary diagnoses, procedures, and discharge status.

Principal diagnosis. Correctly identifying the principal diagnosis is the most important factor in DRG assignment. The principal diagnosis code is the first code listed on the hospital claim and is defined as "that condition established after study to be chiefly responsible for occasioning the admission of the patient to the hospital for care."

On average, 70% of patients are assigned to a medical DRG where changing the principal diagnosis will usually impact the DRG; surgical DRGs are primarily driven by the surgical procedure and not the principal diagnosis.

Secondary diagnoses. All other conditions, either present on admission or that develop subsequently, may qualify as secondary diagnoses if they affect patient care. CMS has designated certain conditions as CCs (comorbidities or complications) and MCCs (major CCs) that may affect MS-DRG assignment:

- **Complication/comorbidity (CC).** A condition in MS-DRGs that
  contributes to the severity of illness and complexity of care of
  patients and often enhances the relative weight of a DRG.
  - Comorbidity. A preexisting condition that affects the treatment
    received and/or increases the length of stay by at least one day
    in approximately 75% of cases.
  - Complication. A condition arising during the hospital stay that
    prolongs the length of stay by at least one day in approximately
    75% of the cases.
- **Major CC (MCC).** A condition in MS-DRGs that contributes to
  substantially greater severity of illness and complexity of care
  than simple CCs and can dramatically enhance the relative
  weight of most DRGs.

Non-CC	CC	MCC
Altered mental status	Delirium due to Xanax withdrawal	Toxic Encephalopathy
Severe COPD on Home O2	Chronic Respiratory Failure	Acute on Chronic Respiratory Failure
Cystitis	Acute cystitis UTI	Sepsis due to UTI
Angina or CAD	Unstable Angina CAD of CABG graft	NSTEMI
CHF	Systolic CHF Diastolic CHF	Acute Systolic CHF Acute Diastolic CHF

Sometimes a diagnosis usually designated as an MCC or CC may
be excluded with certain DRGs when the MCC or CC is too closely
related to the principal diagnosis. For example, CKD stage 5 is a CC;
however when used with a principal diagnosis of acute renal failure,
the CC is excluded from impacting the MS-DRG; it does not "count."

Procedures. All significant procedures are to be reported. UHDDS
defines significant procedures as those that are surgical in nature,
carry a procedural risk, carry an anesthetic risk, or require specialized

training. Most of these are classified as "O.R." procedures that affect DRG assignment. Procedures that do not affect the DRG are considered "non-O.R." such as colonoscopy or bronchial biopsy.

Discharge status. A two-digit code is required on claims to report the patient's discharge disposition (e.g., home, AMA, transferred, expired) that can impact DRG assignment or reimbursement. When the discharge disposition code indicates the patient was discharged with continuing healthcare services (e.g., acute care hospital transfer, skilled nursing facility admission, home health services) the hospital's MS-DRG reimbursement may be reduced (see *GMLOS* above).

Point of origin for admission. The Point of Origin for Admission or Visit Code is reported on the billing claim, indicates the source of the referral for the admission or visit and is essential for accurate reporting. For example, patients admitted from hospice care and who expired may be excluded from certain mortality measures.

Ethical standards. The American Health Information Management Association (AHIMA) and the American Academy of Professional Coders (AAPC) have published standards for ethical coding. The Association of Clinical Documentation Integrity Specialists (ACDIS) has also published a Code of Ethics for documentation specialists. These standards prohibit misrepresentation of the patient's clinical picture through improper coding to increase reimbursement, justify medical necessity, improve publicly reported data, or qualify for insurance policy coverage benefits.

Coding of complications of care can be challenging. The following is an effort to provide a consistent approach to accurately assign codes for complications of care.

GENERAL GUIDELINES

- While conditions classified as complications of care are typically unexpected or unusual outcomes caused by the care rendered, the term "complication" as used in ICD-10 **does not necessarily imply** that improper or inadequate care was provided. Rather, it is important that these are reported to improve patient quality and outcomes.

- Remember that the instructions and conventions of the **ICD-10 classification** take precedence over the Official Coding Guidelines, which take precedence over any other source of coding advice including Coding Clinic. Do not code a condition as a complication from the Index only; veriy the codes in the Tabular.

- Since the **ICD-10 reclassification** of complication of care codes in 2016, in most cases the classification governs code assignment and a causal relationship does not have to be specified.

- Specific **intraoperative** and **postprocedural** complication codes are found at the end of each body system chapter. ICD-10 categories T80-T88 are for complications of medical and surgical care that are not specific to a body system.

- **No time limit** is defined for the development of a complication of care. It may occur during the hospital episode in which the care was provided, shortly thereafter, or even years later.

- Don't become **encoder-dependent**. Terminology in the Index or Tabular List of ICD-10 will often provide insight or guidance for code assignment. Also check Includes and Excludes notes.

- Whenever there is doubt, confusion, disagreement, or conflicting information about the correct interpretation of documentation in the medical record, query the provider.

SPECIFIC GUIDELINES

Official Coding Guidelines Section I.B.16, Documentation of Complications of Care: "Code assignment is based on the provider's documentation of the relationship between the condition and the care or procedure, **unless otherwise instructed by the classification.** The guideline extends to any complications of care, regardless of the chapter the code is located in. It is important to note that not all conditions that occur during or following medical care or surgery are classified as complications. There must be a cause-and-effect relationship between the care provided and the condition, and an indication in the documentation that it is a complication. Query the provider for clarification, if the complication is not clearly documented."

For complications and disorders that are "implicit" or occur during a specific "time period" (e.g., intraoperative, postprocedural), the provider does not have to establish a causal relationship since code assignment is "instructed by the classification."

Complications and disorders that are "implicit" include postoperative infection, postoperative hemorrhage, and complications and disorders of implanted devices.

The Index and Tabular instructional terms "intraoperative," "postprocedural," "postsurgical," "during a procedure," and "following a procedure" in most circumstances indicate that the condition is classified as a complication without further clarification.

Examples include:

- Surgical wound infection following hernia repair (T81.40XA)
- Surgical wound dehiscence (T81.31XA)
- Postprocedural pneumothorax (J95.811)
- Intraoperative cardiac arrest during CABG (I97.710)
- Hematoma following cardiac catheterization (I97.630)
- Postprocedural hemorrhage of the spleen following a splenic procedure (D78.21)
- Rib fractures due to CPR (M96.89)

- Leakage of cystostomy catheter (T83.030A)
- Kidney transplant rejection (T86.11)

Alternatively, where the ICD-10 classification does not include the terms intraoperative or postoperative for a specific condition or includes the terms "resulting from," "due to," or "complicating" a procedure, the provider must specify a causal relationship. Examples include:

- **Intraoperative hemorrhage during CABG** is not coded to (I97.411) "intraoperative hemorrhage of a circulatory system organ *complicating* cardiac bypass" unless there is an indication in the documentation that it is a complication. However, if the hemorrhage is due to accidental puncture/laceration it would be assigned complication code I97.51 "accidental puncture and laceration to a circulatory system organ during a circulatory system procedure" without a need for establishing a causal relationship.

- **Postprocedural subcutaneous emphysema** is not coded to T81.82XA "Emphysema *resulting from* a procedure" unless a causal relationship is established.

- **Postoperative atrial fibrillation** is coded only as atrial fibrillation (I48.91) unless the physician specifies that it is a complication. Documentation of "CABG complicated by postoperative atrial fibrillation" would be coded to I97.89 "Other postprocedural *complications* of the circulatory system NEC," followed by I48.91 "atrial fibrillation."

- **Postoperative ileus** is assigned code K56.7 (ileus), unless the physician specifically confirms that the postoperative ileus is a complication. If specified as a complication, it would be coded to K91.89 "Other postprocedural complications of the digestive system" with K56.7 assigned as an additional code.

Other conditions that occur postoperatively and reported when documented include, for example, postprocedural fever (R50.82), postprocedural peritoneal adhesions (K66.0), postoperative pain (G89.18).

Exceptions include:

- Conditions occurring during **pregnancy** are assumed to affect the pregnancy. It is the provider's responsibility to state that the condition being treated is not affecting the pregnancy.

- For **intraoperative and postoperative CVA** (I97.81-, I97.82-), OCG I.C.9.c states that "medical record documentation must clearly specify the cause-and-effect relationship between the medical intervention and the cerebrovascular accident," even though the ICD-10 classification indicates otherwise.

- **Postprocedural respiratory failure**: See *Respiratory Failure—Postprocedural* in this guide.

Transplant Complications. Transplant complication and rejection are coded under category T86, Complications of transplanted organs and tissues. A transplant complication code is assigned only if the complication affects the function of the transplanted organ. Use two codes to describe the transplant complication: category T86 and another for the specific complication. Pre-existing conditions or conditions that develop after the transplant are not coded as complications unless they affect the function of the transplanted organ.

> **EXAMPLE** A bilateral lung transplant patient admitted with aspiration pneumonia would be coded as T86.818, Other complications of lung transplant, with code J69.0, Aspiration pneumonia. The aspiration pneumonia has affected the function of the transplanted lung.

Complications of **kidney transplant** should only be assigned for documented complications of the kidney transplant, such as failure or rejection or other transplant complication such as AKI. The presence of CKD alone does not constitute a transplant complication since by definition all kidney transplant patients have CKD.

References

- ICD-10-CM Classification
- Official Coding Guidelines, Sections I.B.16, I.C.19.g, and I.C.9.c
- Coding Clinic 2017 First Quarter p. 40
- Coding Clinic 2019 Second Quarter p. 22.

The Affordable Care Act of 2010 mandated the development of quality reporting and pay for performance programs in all practice settings including hospitals, outpatient facilities, physician practices and post-acute care.

The hospital and physician pay for performance (P4P) programs support CMS' goal of improving health care for Medicare fee-for-service (FFS) beneficiaries by linking payment to the quality of hospital care. These are different from the Medicare Star Rating System used to measure how well Medicare Advantage plans perform.

HOSPITAL P4P PROGRAMS

There are three CMS hospital P4P programs in which all hospitals (who serve Medicare FFS patients) participate:

1. Hospital Value-Based Purchasing Program
2. Hospital Readmissions Reduction Program
3. Hospital-Acquired Condition Reduction Program

All three P4P programs include measures that are risk-adjusted based on certain comorbid conditions. The specific measures that are risk adjusted include mortality rates, THA/TKA complication rates, read-mission rates, Medicare spending per beneficiary (MSPB), and PSI-90.

In August 2021, CMS finalized a policy under which CMS can suppress (i.e., not use) measure data for the three hospital P4P programs if it is determined that circumstances caused by the COVID-19 public health emergency have affected those measures and the resulting quality scores significantly.

The three hospital P4P programs are described below.

Hospital Value-Based Purchasing (VBP) Program is a budget-neutral program funded by reducing hospitals base operating DRG payments each fiscal year by 2% and redistributing the entire amount back to the hospitals as value-based incentive payments based on patient care, quality, cost efficiency, and patient satisfaction measures. The amount each hospital receives depends on its ranking compared with all other hospitals.

A hospital with average performance gets back the 2% withheld (a net change of zero). Those below average get back less than the 2% withheld (0% back for the very worst performance—a net loss of 2%). The best performers get back an additional amount up to 2% above the 2% withheld. Therefore, the risk/opportunity ranges between −2% to +2% of DRG payments.

The 2022 VBP consists of four components (domains) of equal weight (25% each) that include a total of 20 measures:

1. **Clinical Outcomes:** 30-day mortality rates for acute MI, heart failure, COPD, pneumonia, CABG; THA/TKA complication rate.

2. **Person and Community Engagement:** 8 measures of patient satisfaction from the Hospital Consumer Assessment of Healthcare Providers and Systems (HCAHPS) survey.

3. **Efficiency and Cost Reduction:** Medicare Spending Per Beneficiary (MSPB) = all Part A and B payments to all providers from 3 days prior to admission through 30 days post discharge.

4. **Safety**: CLABSI, CAUTI, CDI (Clostridium difficile infection), MRSA bacteremia, SSI (surgical site infections) for abdominal hysterectomy and colon surgery.

The Clinical Outcomes and Efficiency and Cost Reduction component measures are risk-adjusted based on certain comorbid conditions.

For FY 2022, CMS will suppress most hospital VBP Program measures resulting in hospitals receiving neutral payment adjustments for FY 2022.

Hospital Readmissions Reduction Program (HRRP). The HRRP reduces payments to hospitals with excess readmissions of Medicare patients 65 years of age or older originally admitted ("index admission") with any of four diagnoses (acute MI, heart failure, pneumonia, COPD) or two procedures (CABG and elective hip or knee replacement).

A readmission is defined as a patient who is readmitted for any reason to the same or another acute care hospital within 30 days of discharge. The 30-day readmission measure excludes planned readmissions, such as planned chemotherapy or rehabilitation.

The excess readmission rate for each of the six index admission categories is defined as exceeding the risk-adjusted national average readmission rate. The total penalty is an aggregate of any penalties for each of the six categories. The maximum penalty is 3% each year.

As noted before, the severity of illness based on certain comorbid conditions influences the risk adjustment for the readmission rates. Sicker patients are expected to have higher readmission rates, so hospitals with a patient population reflecting higher severity of illness will have their readmission rates adjusted downward and therefore are less likely to be penalized.

For FY 2023, CMS will suppress the pneumonia readmissions measure and exclude COVID-19 patients from the remaining five measures.

Hospital-Acquired Condition Reduction Program (HACRP). The HACRP creates an incentive for hospitals to reduce certain hospital-acquired conditions by reducing payment by 1% for those hospitals that rank in the worst performing quartile (worst 25%). The 2022 HACRP comprises (1) CMS PSI 90 and (2) CDC hospital acquired infections.

(1) CMS PSI 90: Includes a composite of the below ten "claims-based" Patient Safety Indicators (PSIs). These are derived from ICD-10 codes with POA status assigned on the hospital claim and determined by physician documentation.

- PSI-03 Pressure ulcer (17%)
- PSI-06 Iatrogenic pneumothorax (4%)
- PSI-08 In-hospital fall with hip fracture (1%)
- PSI-09 Perioperative hemorrhage or hematoma (5%)
- PSI-10 Postoperative acute kidney injury requiring dialysis (8%)
- PSI-11 Postoperative respiratory failure (16%)
- PSI-12 Perioperative pulmonary embolism or DVT (19%)
- PSI-13 Postoperative sepsis (25%)

- PSI-14 Postoperative wound dehiscence (<1%)
- PSI-15 Unrecognized abdominopelvic accidental puncture/ laceration (4%)

*Note that **four measures** (pressure ulcer, postoperative respiratory failure, periopera- tive PE/DVT, postoperative sepsis) contribute 77% to the total PSI-90 measure score.*

(2) CDC Hospital Acquired Infection (HAI) measures: Derived from "abstracted" measures for adverse events. Measure abstraction is typ- ically performed by a hospital's quality or infection control depart- ment using CDC case definitions based on objective information in the medical record independent of physician documentation. Physi- cian documentation and code assignment have no influence on these abstracted measures. The six measures are:

- CLABSI (central line–associated bloodstream infection)
- CAUTI (catheter-associated UTI)
- SSI (surgical site infections) for total hysterectomy and colon surgery
- MRSA bacteremia (positive blood culture)
- Clostridium difficile infection

Each measure for which a hospital has a measure score is of equal weight. For example, if a hospital only has a measure score for PSI-90, CLABSI, CAUTI, MRSA bacteremia, and C-diff infection (5 of the 6 measures), each measure would account for 20% (1/5) of the total measure score.

CMS will exclude performance data from 2020 in calculating the HAC Reduction Program performance for FYs 2022 and 2023.

HAC DRG Penalty (Deficit Reduction Act). This HAC penalty program is not a P4P program but has been in place since 2009. A patient discharge is not assigned to a higher-paying DRG if certain HAC conditions are not POA, i.e., they are excluded as MCC/CCs, although if another MCC/ CC is included on the claim no payment adjustment is made. There are 14 categories of conditions, including stage 3/4 pressure ulcers, foreign objects retained after surgery, ABO incompatibility, iatrogenic pneumothorax, etc.

PHYSICIAN P4P PROGRAMS

Like hospitals, clinicians are incentivized to improve quality of care and reduce costs through the CMS Quality Payment Program. These quality incentive programs for physicians and other eligible clinicians reward value and outcomes through Alternative Payment Models (APMs) and the Merit-based Incentive Payment System (MIPS).

An Alternative Payment Model (APM) is a payment approach that gives added incentive payments to encourage high-quality and cost-efficient care. The different models can apply to a specific clinical condition, a care episode, or a population. APM examples include joint replacement (bundled payments), comprehensive ESRD care, accountable care organizations (ACO), among others.

Accountable Care Organizations (ACOs). ACOs are groups of healthcare providers (physicians and hospitals) that agree to be accountable for the cost and quality of care for a group of beneficiaries. For this defined population of beneficiaries, Medicare ACOs are "accountable" for the total Medicare Part A and Part B spending and their quality of care.

Providers in ACOs continue to be paid their normal fee-for-service rates but can earn bonus payments if at the end of the year actual total spending is less than the expected spending (based on a predetermined benchmark) for those beneficiaries. If there is a savings (actual spending is less than expected), those savings are shared between Medicare and the ACO at a defined shared savings rate. The calculation of savings and losses are influenced by their quality measures and beneficiary risk adjustment scores based on HCCs. The higher the quality and risk scores the greater share of the savings the ACO receives.

Merit-based Incentive Payment System. The vast majority of clinicians currently participate in MIPS. MIPS was designed to tie payments to quality and cost-efficient care, drive improvement in care processes and health outcomes, increase the use of healthcare information, and reduce the cost of care.

MIPS determines traditional Medicare fee schedule adjustments. Using a composite performance score, eligible clinicians may receive a payment bonus, penalty or no payment adjustment. The potential MIPS adjustment for CY and beyond +/−9% for 2022. The 2020 performance period will determine the 2022 adjustment.

MIPS eligible clinicians include physicians, physician assistants, nurse practitioners, clinical nurse specialists, and certified registered nurse anesthetists.

In response to the COVID-19 public health emergency, CMS is implementing multiple flexibilities for the Quality Payment Program, resulting in the reweighting of many of the performance year measures below.

The 2022 MIPS performance year score will be based on the following measures:

1. **Quality—30%**

   Clinicians must collect and submit data for at least 6 measures selected from a list of 195 proposed measures; at least one must be an Outcome measure.

   Examples of measures include: Age appropriate screening colonoscopy, 30-day all-cause hospital readmission rate, controlling high blood pressure, biopsy follow-up, breast cancer screening, zoster (shingles) vaccination.

2. **Cost—30%**
   - Medicare spending per beneficiary measure (MSPB)
   - Total per capita costs for all attributed beneficiaries (TPCC)
   - 13 episode-based cost measures, e.g., knee arthroplasty, elective outpatient PCI, screening colonoscopy, simple pneumonia with hospitalization.

3. Promoting Interoperability—25%

Data must be collected and submitted for each of four objectives from a list of 40 proposed measures for 90 continuous days or more during 2021. Examples include E-prescribing, immunization registry reporting, patient electronic access, security risk analysis. *This replaced the EHR incentive established in 2011.*

4. Improvement Activities—15%

Clinicians must submit activities selected from a list of 119 measures (based on a specified combination of low, medium, and high-weighted activities) and performed for 90 continuous days or more during 2021.

Examples of measures include: depression screening, diabetes screening, unhealthy alcohol use, advance care planning, engagement of patients through implementation of improvements in patient portal, anticoagulant management improvements.

Although most of these measures are not risk-adjusted, some of the quality measures such as the 30-day readmission rate and cost measures are risk-adjusted based on the codes submitted on Part A and Part B claims using HCC diagnoses.

References

- CMS Quality Payment Program: www.qpp.cms.gov
- Accountable Care Payment Systems, MedPac, October 2018.

To understand HCCs, it is helpful to first understand the differences between traditional fee-for-service (FFS) Medicare and Medicare Advantage. **Traditional FFS Medicare** includes Part A (inpatient care) and Part B (outpatient services), and benefits are paid directly from the federal government (CMS) to providers. Traditional Medicare health benefits are the same for every person who enrolls and offers more flexibility than a Medicare Advantage plan; for example, you can use any healthcare provider who accepts Medicare and prior authorization for services is not required.

Another Medicare health plan is Medicare Part C, **Medicare Advantage**. CMS allows private health insurers to set up managed care plans to cover Medicare beneficiaries. As of 2021, 42 percent of Medicare-eligible beneficiaries are enrolled in a Medicare Advantage plan. CMS pays the insurer a monthly fixed capitation rate for each beneficiary enrolled as a member of a Medicare Advantage (MA) plan. MA plans must then use that money to pay hospitals, physicians, and other health care providers for the services the plan members receive.

While all MA plans must cover the same services as Parts A and B, many MA plans offer additional covered services that traditional Medicare does not such as vision, hearing, dental. However, MA plans typically require members to choose a primary care provider within their network, referrals to see specialists, and prior authorization for procedures and services.

What are HCCs? Hierarchical Condition Categories, or HCCs, were originally developed by CMS as a payment methodology for Medicare Advantage (MA) plans. The CMS-HCC payment methodology enables CMS to forecast costs for MA plan members for the coming year by calculating anticipated "risk" from certain ICD-10 diagnosis codes, which are primarily chronic conditions. MA plans are paid a fixed amount (per member/per month) to cover the healthcare costs of their members based on the prior year's risk adjustment score: higher payments for sicker populations, lower payments for healthier populations.

Diagnostic information submitted on claims directly affects the payments an MA health plan receives for each of its MA members by influencing a patient's risk score, i.e., risk adjustment factor (RAF). Therefore, CMS payments to MA plans are *directly* affected by the number of HCC diagnosis codes assigned on the encounter.

On the other hand, hospitals and providers continue to bill and be paid using the same fee-for-service model currently in place (inpatient DRG, CPT code, etc.) for both traditional Medicare (by CMS) and Medicare Advantage patients (by the MA health plan). However, certain HCC (and MCC/CC) conditions are used to risk-adjust some of the cost and quality measures included in the hospital CMS pay-for-performance programs for the traditional Medicare patient population. Performance in these programs can impact the overall hospital FFS DRG payment rate which is adjusted to reward outcomes believed to indicate higher-quality care and penalize outcomes thought to indicate lower-quality care.

In addition, Medicare payments to providers and Accountable Care Organizations (ACOs) based on quality and cost-saving measures are risk-adjusted based on certain HCC conditions. In both these cases, payments to the hospital or physician are *indirectly* affected by HCCs which is why HCC capture has become a focus for hospitals and physician practices. See ***CMS Pay for Performance Programs***.

HCC payment methodologies. The two primary HCC methodologies are (1) CMS-HCCs for Medicare Advantage (Part C) plans and (2) Health and Human Services (HHS-HCC) for managed commercial health plans as part of the Affordable Care Act. Medicare Advantage plans have been paid by CMS based on CMS-HCCs since 2004, and managed commercial health plans based on HHS-HCCs since 2014.

There are a number of other risk adjustment payment methodologies that have been developed since the HCC models including CDPS (Chronic Illness and Disability Payment System) primarily used for Medicaid managed care plans and DxCG (Diagnostic Cost Groups) used by other commercial managed care plans.

CMS-HCC payment methodology for MA plans. CMS-HCCs include approximately 9,500 diagnosis codes, of which 5,500 are MCCs/CCs and 4,000 are chronic non-CC conditions. Common HCCs that are non-CCs include: COPD/emphysema, dementia, diabetic complications, morbid obesity, rheumatoid arthritis, amputation status and artificial openings.

The HCC system determines a patient's risk adjustment factor (RAF) based on ICD-10 diagnosis codes (like inpatient DRGs). HCC categories are designed to group conditions that are clinically similar and follow similar cost patterns to predict future healthcare costs.

Each HCC carries a risk adjustment coefficient or weight, like the DRG relative weight, and contains from one to several hundred diagnostic codes.

Example of CMS-HCCs and Weights

HCC	HCC Description	# of Codes	Weight V24.0
1	HIV/AIDS	3	0.344
2	Septicemia, Sepsis, SIRS/Shock	51	0.428
6	Opportunistic Infections	37	0.446
8	Metastatic Cancer and Acute Leukemia	81	2.654

An HCC's value reflects the cost, complexity and severity of the conditions it contains. HCC conditions and weights are primarily driven by chronic diseases, which tend to have greater annual costs than episodes of acute conditions.

Note: The CMS-HCC versions are not updated annually like MS-DRGs.

The CMS-HCC risk adjustment payment model, which determines payment for MA payors (not providers), uses an individual's demographic data and HCC diagnoses from the prior year to determine a risk score — a relative measure of how costly that individual's care is anticipated to be — for the subsequent year.

Risk scores are reset to 0 in January each year — and the HCC slate is wiped clean. All chronic non-resolving HCC diagnoses and any new diagnoses need to be reported at least once during the calendar year.

A total weight of 1.0 represents an individual with average annual costs. A higher weight represents a sicker patient with higher costs and a higher payment. Conversely, a lower weight indicates a healthier, less costly patient with a lower payment.

For diseases that are not closely related, HCCs are cumulative (added up); for example, a patient with CKD, heart failure, and cancer, will have those three respective HCCs added together. However, each single HCC can be used only once during the calendar year for the calculation of the risk score.

Each MA member's **RAF** is based on demographic criteria and their HCC diagnoses for the prior year and used to calculate a per member per month payment to the MA payor in the subsequent year. The health plan is "at risk" if the healthcare costs for the individual exceeds the monthly payment.

The table below illustrates the CMS-HCC risk adjustment factor (RAF) scoring for a hypothetical patient in an **MA plan**, using both the patient's demographics and the information in the medical record:

Description	HCC	Weight
80 year old male, community, aged	Demographics	0.540
Angina (I20.9)	88	0.143
Diabetes (E11.9)	19	0.106
Pneumonia (J18.9)	-	0.0
Acute respiratory failure (J96.00)	84	0.314
Total RAF		1.103
Annual payment		$11,030

The annual payment of $11,030 is based on this patient's total RAF x a plan base payment rate of $10,000 (1.103 x $10,000).

For CY2022 CMS will calculate MA risk scores used for payment based entirely on MA encounter data and Medicare fee-for-service (FFS) claims as the sources of diagnoses. Therefore, hospitals and physicians who are better at capturing relevant HCC diagnosis codes thereby directly increase the amount that CMS reimburses the MA health plan. This explains why many insurance companies encourage hospitals and physicians to document HCCs. Nevertheless, there are indirect benefits for hospitals and physicians who have pay-for-performance or value-based agreements since proper documentation of certain HCC conditions could influence some quality and cost measures and subsequent incentive payments.

HCC capture in the inpatient setting. Capture of certain HCC diagnoses can affect risk-adjustment of some of the quality and outcome measures (mortality, readmission rates) included in the CMS Pay for Performance programs, which for the most part are based primarily on inpatient data.

To incorporate HCCs into your inpatient CDI review process, first optimize the MS-DRG assignment with identification of MCC/CCs and APR-DRG severity levels. Most diagnoses that influence APR-DRG severity are also CCs or MCCs; there are only a few non-CC conditions that can change the APR-DRG severity level. On the other hand, HCCs tend to be chronic conditions and over half of the CMS-HCCs are CCs or MCCs. For example, a metastatic cancer diagnosis which is a CC is the highest-weighted HCC and significantly affects risk adjustment for most quality measures. This should be a CDI focus to ensure this diagnosis (when supported) is always coded on the claim.

The CDI team should make a list of the more common, high-impact HCC diagnoses to ensure capture and query for these diagnoses as well. The *Comorbid Condition* section that includes the CMS-HCC list in this guide will help you identify your focus list.

"Present on admission" means present at the time the order for inpatient admission occurs. Conditions considered present on admission include any that occur in the emergency department, observation, clinic, or outpatient surgery prior to the inpatient admission.

POA INDICATORS:

- **Y** (Yes): Present at the time of inpatient admission

- **N** (No): Not present at the time of inpatient admission

- **U** (Unknown): Documentation is insufficient to determine if condition is present on admission (MD should be queried), and equivalent to a N (No).

- **W** (Clinically undetermined): Provider is unable to clinically determine whether condition was present on admission or not, and equivalent to Y (Yes).

- **I** (Unreported/not used): Exempt from POA reporting.

CONDITIONS THAT ARE PRESENT ON ADMISSION

- Conditions explicitly documented as being present on admission

- Conditions that were diagnosed prior to admission (heart failure, diabetes, COPD)

- Conditions diagnosed during the admission that were clearly present but not diagnosed until after admission occurred (e.g., patient with lung nodule is admitted, has a biopsy and pathology reveals lung carcinoma)

- Diagnoses subsequently confirmed after admission if at the time of admission they are documented as suspected, possible, rule out, differential diagnosis, or **constitute an underlying cause of a symptom** that is present at the time of admission

- A final diagnosis that contains a possible, probable, suspected, or rule out diagnosis, and this diagnosis was based on symptoms or clinical findings suspected at the time of inpatient admission

- Conditions assigned to codes that contain multiple clinical concepts and all parts of a combination code were present on admission, e.g., duodenal ulcer that perforates prior to admission; patient admitted with ruptured aortic aneurysm

- Any external cause code representing an external cause of morbidity that occurred prior to admission, e.g., patient fell out of bed at home.

POA Documentation. Medical record documentation from any provider involved in the care and treatment of the patient may be used to support the determination of whether a condition was present on admission. The term "provider" means a physician or any qualified healthcare practitioner who is legally accountable for establishing the patient's diagnosis.

Disease severity and progression. For conditions that are present on admission that progress during a stay (except pressure ulcers), only one code is assigned to capture the highest level of severity with POA status=Y. For example, mild preeclampsia that progresses to severe, or moderate malnutrition that progresses to severe.

Per Coding Clinic 2020 First Quarter, p. 4: OCG I.C.12.b.3 *"specifically applies to pressure ulcers in order to track the change in stage during an inpatient admission and is not intended to be applied to other conditions."*

CMS has no **limitation** on the time period during which a provider must identify or document that a condition was present on admission.

Reference
- Official Coding Guidelines, Appendix I: Present on Admission Reporting Guidelines

ICD-10 has directions that require a certain code to be assigned when two conditions are related. Terms to indicate what these associations are include "with," "associated with," "in," and "due to."

OCG provides guidance in Section I.A.15 (titled "With"): "The word 'with' or 'in' should be interpreted to mean 'associated with' or 'due to' when it appears in a code title, the Alphabetic Index, or an instructional note in the Tabular List. The classification **presumes a causal relationship between the two conditions** linked by these terms in the Alphabetic Index or Tabular List. These conditions should be coded as related even in the absence of provider documentation explicitly linking them, **unless the documentation clearly states the conditions are unrelated.** For conditions not specifically linked by these relational terms in the classification, provider documentation must link the conditions in order to code them as related, or when another guideline exists that specifically requires a documented linkage between two conditions (e.g., sepsis guidelines for 'acute organ dysfunction that is not clearly associated with the sepsis')."

All of the **diabetic complications** listed in the ICD-10 Index (except those indexed as "NEC") are automatically linked (e.g., neuropathy, retinopathy, gangrene, gastroparesis, osteomyelitis) and the diabetic code can be assigned. If listed as an NEC code, the causal relationship must be established by the provider. See ***Diabetic Complications***.

The "With" rule also presumes a causal relationship between gastric ulcer and **GI bleeding** (unless another cause of GI bleeding is specified), and therefore logically applies to any GI condition having a code for "with hemorrhage." See Coding Clinic 2017 Third Quarter, p. 27.

The link between **hypertension and heart disease** is assumed as a causal relationship (same as hypertension and kidney involvement), and the provider no longer has to specify the connection.

If it appears from the record that a related condition might not be due to the other but rather caused by another condition, it is prudent to seek clarification even though the classification and OCG do not require it.

Signs and symptoms. A "sign" is objective evidence of disease observed by examining the patient. A "symptom" is a subjective observation reported by the patient. A "diagnosis" is a statement of conclusion that describes the reason for a disease, illness, or problem.

Misperceptions associated with the coding of signs and symptoms can be a source of coding errors. The coding guidelines discourage assigning codes for signs and symptoms instead of a diagnosis.

Signs and symptoms are classified in ICD-10 Chapter 18 (R00-R99) and include abnormal clinical and laboratory findings.

"Codes that describe symptoms and signs, as opposed to diagnoses, are acceptable for reporting purposes when a related definitive diagnosis has ***not been established*** (confirmed) by the provider." (OCG I.B.4).

"Signs and symptoms that are associated routinely with a disease process should not be assigned as additional codes, unless otherwise instructed by the classification." (OCG I.B.5).

"Additional signs and symptoms that may not be associated routinely with a disease process should be coded when present." (OCG I.B.6).

The determination of what signs and symptoms are "routinely associated with" every disease process encountered is sometimes challenging. This does not constitute "interpretation of the medical record," but requires coding professionals to be familiar with the signs and symptoms of disease processes.

"Signs and symptoms ***are not to be used as principal diagnosis*** when a related definitive diagnosis has been established." (OCG II.A).

Signs and symptoms associated with a primary or secondary site malignancy cannot be used to replace the malignancy as the principal or first-listed diagnosis, regardless of the number of admissions or encounters for treatment and care of the neoplasm (OCG I.C.2.g).

Per the instructional note at the beginning of Chapter 18, the situations in which the conditions and signs and symptoms included in categories R00-R94 would be appropriately assigned are:

"(a) cases for which no more specific diagnosis can be made even after all the facts bearing on the case have been investigated;

(b) signs or symptoms existing at the time of initial encounter that proved to be transient and whose causes could not be determined;

(c) provisional diagnosis in a patient who failed to return for further investigation or care;

(d) cases referred elsewhere for investigation or treatment before the diagnosis was made;

(e) cases in which a more precise diagnosis was not available for any other reason;

(f) certain symptoms, for which supplementary information is provided, that represent important problems in medical care in their own right."

Unspecified codes. For inpatients, codes are assigned to the highest degree of specificity documented by providers in the medical record, including uncertain diagnoses (those documented as probable, suspected, likely, etc.). According to CMS: "When sufficient clinical information isn't known or available about a particular health condition to assign a more specific code, it is acceptable to report the appropriate 'unspecified' code."

Therefore, when a documented diagnosis results in an unspecified code, a query is needed only when a more specific code impacts DRG assignment, risk adjustment, pay for performance measures, or helps to justify medical necessity. ***Documentation of greater specificity by providers is not necessary simply because a more specific code exists.***

OCG I.A.9.b. instructs coders to limit the use of unspecified codes as follows: "Codes titled 'unspecified' are for use when information in the medical record is insufficient to assign a more specific code. For those categories for which an unspecified code is not provided, the 'other specified' code may represent both other and unspecified."

"Sign/symptom and 'unspecified' codes have acceptable, even necessary, uses. While specific diagnosis codes should be reported when they are supported by the available medical record documentation and clinical knowledge of the patient's health condition, there are instances when signs/symptoms or unspecified codes are the best choices for accurately reflecting the healthcare encounter. Each healthcare encounter should be coded to the level of certainty known for that encounter." (OCG I.B.18)

Unspecified, or NOS, codes should not be assigned when more specific detail is documented in the medical record. The medical record should be searched carefully for any additional information that might permit assignment of a more specific code, thereby giving a more accurate and complete account of the patient's condition and treatment.

For example, congestive heart failure, unspecified (I50.9) is a commonly assigned unspecified code. Finding documentation of systolic and/or diastolic failure and the acuity anywhere in the medical record by a provider should permit assignment of the correct and most specific codes. If the necessary information isn't there, a query would be appropriate.

According to AHIMA, social determinants of health (SDOH) are "the economic, social, and behavioral conditions that influence the health and quality of life of individuals and populations."

Codes describing social determinants of health (SDOH) should be assigned when this information is documented.

SDOH code categories Z55-Z65 include:
- Homelessness (Z59.00)
- Extreme poverty (Z59.5):
- Imprisonment and other incarceration (Z65.1)
- Alcoholism and drug addiction in family (Z63.72)

Coding professionals may utilize non-physician documentation of social information from social workers, community health workers, case managers, or nurses, if their documentation is included in the official medical record. It is also appropriate to utilize patient self-reported documentation if it is signed-off and incorporated into the medical record by either a clinician or provider.

Although these codes do not currently impact DRG assignment, risk adjustment or pay for performance, there are a number of national initiatives such as one of CMS' innovation models "Accountable Health Communities" which is assessing whether addressing health-related social needs through enhanced clinical-community collaboration can improve health outcomes and reduce costs. Unmet health-related social needs may increase the risk of developing chronic conditions, reduce an individual's ability to manage these conditions, increase health care costs, and lead to avoidable health care utilization.

References:
- OCG I.C.21.c.17: Social Determinants of Health
- CMS Accountable Health Communities Model
- AHIMA White Paper: SDOH: Improving Capture and Use by Applying Data Governance Strategies

CMS deferred the promulgation of specific guidelines addressing query practices to health information management experts and organizations. In its 2001 policy statement regarding queries, CMS "allows the use of the physician query to the extent it provides clarification and is consistent with other medical record documentation." Healthcare facilities can "adapt these forms to meet their individual needs" and "recognize that flexibility is necessary to allow this individualized adaptation to occur."

The 2019 AHIMA/ACDIS "Guidelines for Achieving a Compliant Query Practice" provides industry-wide best practices for the query function and includes these basic "tenets" for a compliant query:

- Queries must be accompanied by clinical indicator(s) that are specific to the patient and episode of care and support why a more complete or accurate diagnosis or procedure is sought.

- Avoid queries that:
    - Fail to include clinical indicators that justify the query or justify the choices provided within a multiple-choice format
    - Encourage, suggest or lead the provider to a specific diagnosis or procedure
    - Indicate the impact on reimbursement, payment methodology, or quality metrics
    - Include terms that indicate an "uncertain" diagnosis as a query response choice (unless the query is provided at the time of discharge or after discharge).

It also states that all queries, whether written or verbal, should be clear and concise, contain clinical indicators from the health record, present only the facts identifying why the clarification is required, and be compliant with the practices outlined in the brief.

WHEN TO QUERY?

Query when there is **conflicting, incomplete, or ambiguous** information in the health record regarding a significant reportable condition or procedure. However, AHIMA/ACDIS 2019 states: "Queries are not necessary for every discrepancy or unaddressed issue in physician documentation." It is critical that facilities balance the value of gaining marginal data quality benefits against the administrative burden of obtaining additional documentation as well as physician query fatigue.

Queries should be made for greater specificity of ICD-10 codes only to support correct DRG assignment or for accurate quality/performance measures. If there is no DRG or quality/performance impact, greater specificity isn't necessary and a query is *not* needed.

Queries should not be used to question a provider's clinical judgment, but rather to clarify documentation. In situations where the clinical indicators or clinical picture does not appear to support the documentation of a condition or procedure, hospital policies should provide guidance for addressing the issue. See ***Clinical Validation***.

WHOM TO QUERY?

Any physician or other qualified healthcare practitioner who is legally accountable for establishing a patient's diagnosis. The provider must be licensed by his or her state and credentialed by the facility to diagnose and treat patients. This includes attending physician, consultant, specialist, emergency physician, anesthesiologist, CRNA, resident, fellow, physician assistant, podiatrist, nurse practitioner.

When there is conflicting information, the attending physician should be queried since he or she is ultimately responsible for the final diagnoses.

WRITTEN QUERY TYPES

Three query types: (1) open-ended, (2) multiple-choice, and (3) Yes/No.

Open-ended query. These queries provide clinical criteria in the medical record but ask a generalized question about their significance. They can be vague and unclear to physicians.

Multiple-choice query. Standardized multiple-choice clarification/query templates for the most common physician queries have many advantages over free-text, open-ended queries. They are often more clear and precise, which helps the provider to understand the purpose of the query and give a reasoned clinical response.

Multiple-choice queries should have a standardized format, such as the following:

Format	Content Example
Reason for the query	Documentation in the medical record indicates the patient was admitted with dyspnea and "severe COPD on home O2."
Pertinent clinical indicators	The following is also documented in the medical record: • Pulse ox on 4L/min in ER = 91% • Home oxygen at 2L/min • Bicarbonate level on BMP = 42
Clinically significant and reasonable options,* and Other, Not applicable/None of the above	Based on your medical judgment, can you further clarify in the progress notes which, if any, of the following conditions are responsible for these findings: • Acute respiratory failure • Chronic respiratory failure • Acute on chronic respiratory failure • Hypoxia only • Other condition (please specify): • Not applicable/None of the above
Closing	In responding to this request, please exercise your independent professional judgment.

*According to the 2019 ACDIS/AHIMA guidelines, "*Multiple choice query formats should include clinically significant and reasonable options as supported by clinical indicators in the health record, recognizing that there may be only one reasonable option.*"

Yes/no query. Use "yes/no" queries to

- Establish a cause-and-effect relationship between documented conditions such as manifestation/etiology, complications and conditions/diagnostic findings

> This patient was admitted with sepsis and acute kidney injury (AKI).
>
> Based on your medical judgment, can you please clarify if the AKI is related or due to the sepsis?
>
> Other? Not applicable?

- Substantiate or further specify a diagnosis that is already present in the health record

- Resolve conflicting practitioner documentation

> The patient was admitted with fever, chills, WBC 16K, and nonspecific chest x-ray. Dr. Smith diagnosed "pneumonia" and Dr. Jones diagnosed "bronchitis without evidence of pneumonia."
>
> Based on your medical judgment, can you please clarify in the medical record whether you agree with the diagnosis of pneumonia?
>
> Other? Not applicable?

- Confirm present on admission status.

> When this patient was admitted, a nursing note documented a stage 3 sacral pressure ulcer. Provider documentation did not occur until day 3. Coding guidelines do not allow use of nursing notes for present on admission status.
>
> Based on your medical judgment, can you please clarify in the medical record if the pressure ulcer was present on admission?
>
> Clinically undetermined? Other?

Yes/No queries should not be used when only clinical indicators of a condition are present and the condition/diagnosis has yet to be documented.

Verbal queries allow for an informational and educational exchange between CDI and provider. A summary of the verbal query should be recorded in CDI working documents that includes the clinical indicators, options provided, and time and date of the discussion.

Query responses can be documented in the progress notes, discharge summary, on the query form as a part of the formal health record, or as an addendum (with actual date of entry and authentication).

Organizational policies should specifically address a **query retention** period indicating whether the query is part of the patient's permanent health record or stored as a separate business record. If the query form is not part of the health record, the policy should specify where it will be filed and the length of time it will be retained.

Although recommended by many experts, incorporating queries into the **legal medical record** may have undesirable consequences such as unnecessarily focusing attention on a missed diagnosis or a surgeon's reluctance to confirm a significant procedural complication.

Conditions from prior encounters. AHIMA/ACDIS 2019: "Prior encounter information may be referenced in queries for clinical clarification and/or validation if it is clinically pertinent to the present encounter. However, it is inappropriate to "mine" a previous encounter's documentation to generate queries not related to the current encounter." Therefore, clinical data pertinent to the current episode of care from a prior episode may be included in the query citing the source of the information as well as the indicators from the current episode.

References

- CMS Policy Clarification on Coding Compliance. QIP TOPS control number: PRO2001-13
- 2019 ACDIS/AHIMA Guidelines for Achieving a Compliant Query Practice
- Medicare Program Integrity Manual, Section 6.5.3.B
- Coding Clinic 2013 Third Quarter p. 27.

In most circumstances, the diagnosis for which a surgical procedure is performed would be assigned as the principal diagnosis. Although uncommon, there are instances when a procedure is performed that is not related to the principal diagnosis for which DRGs 981-983 and 987-989 (O.R. Procedure Unrelated to Principal Diagnosis) are appropriately assigned.

In these cases, always review the record carefully to determine whether the medical condition (or symptoms of the condition) associated with the principal surgical procedure might have been present on admission and could possibly meet the definition of principal diagnosis.

Circumstances for which assignment to an Unrelated O.R. Procedure DRG would be appropriate:

1. Procedure performed for a diagnosis that was clearly not present on admission
   - Patient admitted for pneumonia and experiences an acute MI two days after admission and coronary stent inserted
   - Patient admitted for UGI bleeding that was cauterized, followed by respiratory failure with intubation and transbronchial lung biopsy

2. Incidental, minor procedure performed for a secondary diagnosis
   - Patient admitted with respiratory failure and inguinal lymph node biopsy was performed

3. Procedure performed for a chronic secondary condition for which the patient was not (or would not have been) admitted to the hospital
   - Patient admitted for acute pulmonary embolus and has an umbilical hernia repair

4. Surgical procedure is for principal diagnosis but DRG logic assigns to Unrelated Procedure DRG
   - Patient with stage IV pressure ulcer admitted for elective diverting colostomy to prevent contamination of the ulcer.

Any healthcare "provider." Documentation in the medical record by any healthcare provider is appropriate for code assignment. The term "provider" includes physicians and "other qualified health care practitioner who is legally accountable for establishing the patient's diagnosis" such as consultants, residents, nurse practitioners, physician assistants, etc. "Legally accountable" includes being licensed by the state and credentialed by the hospital, which may exclude first year interns if they are not licensed yet.

There are some exceptions when code assignment may be based on documentation from **other "clinicians"** who are not the patient's provider, and include BMI, pressure ulcer stage, depth of non-pressure chronic ulcers, Glasgow coma scale, NIH stroke scale, social determinants of health (SDOH), laterality, and blood alcohol level.

In this context "clinicians" refer to healthcare professionals permitted, based on regulatory or accreditation requirements or internal hospital policies, to document in a patient's official medical record.

A dietitian often documents the BMI, a nurse often documents pressure ulcer stages, and an EMT often documents the coma scale. However, an **associated diagnosis** (such as overweight, obesity, pressure ulcer, acute stroke, or alcohol related disorder) must be documented by a provider.

For **SDOH** (code categories Z55-Z65), coding professionals may utilize documentation of social information from social workers, case managers, or nurses if their documentation is included in the official medical record. It is also appropriate to use patient self-reported documentation if it is signed off and incorporated into the medical record by a clinician or provider.

According to Coding Clinic 2004, "Code assignment may be based on other provider documentation (i.e., consultants, residents, anesthesiologists, etc.) as long as there is no **conflicting** information from the attending physician. Medical record documentation from any physician involved in the care and treatment of the patient, including documentation by consulting or emergency physicians, is appropriate for the basis of code assignment. A physician query is not necessary if a physician involved in the care and treatment of the patient has documented a diagnosis and there is no conflicting documentation from another physician. If documentation from different physicians conflicts, seek clarification from the attending physician, as he or she is ultimately responsible for the final diagnosis."

Therefore, the attending physician does not have to confirm a diagnosis by another provider unless it is conflicting. A conflict occurs when two physicians call the same condition two different things. It is important to distinguish between "**conflicting**" and "**more specific.**" For example, pneumonia vs. bronchitis is conflicting and would require a query; pneumonia vs. aspiration pneumonia is more specific and would not.

Discharge Summary. Diagnoses do not have to be documented in the discharge summary to be coded which is often the least reliable source. The coding professional must make sure that medical record documentation supports the principal and secondary diagnoses based on a review of the **entire medical record** to ensure complete and accurate coding.

The Official Coding Guidelines, page 1, states "The entire record should be reviewed to determine the specific reason for the encounter and the conditions treated."

According to "Documentation Guidelines" in Coding Clinic 2000 Second Quarter, p. 17-18:

"When documentation in the medical record is clear and consistent, coders may assign and report codes."

"Documentation is not limited to the face sheet, discharge summary, progress notes, history and physical, or other report designed to capture diagnostic information."

References

- CMS MLN Matters Number: SE1121
- Coding Clinic 2000 Second Quarter p. 17-18
- Coding Clinic 2004 First Quarter p. 18-19
- Coding Clinic 2019 Fourth Quarter p. 66

- Official Coding Guidelines I.B.14: Documentation by Clinicians Other than the Patient's Provider.

DEFINITION

An accidental puncture or laceration is a clinically significant cut, puncture, tear, perforation of a blood vessel, nerve or organ that occurs during a procedure.

Examples:
- Perforation of bladder during sigmoid colon resection
- Laceration of spleen during lysis of small bowel adhesions
- Serosal tears of the bowel due to lysis of adhesions
- Incidental dural tear during spinal surgery
- Traumatic intubation resulting in soft palate injury involving ETT

CODING AND DOCUMENTATION CHALLENGES

In ICD-10, accidental punctures and lacerations that occur during a procedure (intraoperatively) are coded to the specific organ and body system. It is not necessary to query the provider whether it is a "complication" of the procedure.

An accidental puncture and laceration code would be assigned unless the documentation is unclear or the condition does not meet the definition of an **additional diagnosis** (requires clinical evaluation, treatment, etc.).

Traumatic injury codes should not be assigned for injuries that occur during, or as a result of, a medical intervention.

Coding Clinic reinforces these instructions in the following scenarios:

For a **serosal injury** of the small intestine requiring bowel excision, assign code K91.71, Accidental puncture and laceration of a digestive system organ or structure during a digestive system procedure — even if the provider states the tear was "unavoidable during extensive lysis of adhesions, not intraoperative complication." According to Coding Clinic 2021 Second Quarter p. 11, "Although after query the provider indicated the serosal tear was unavoidable, it was clinically significant, as it required further excision, complicating the surgery."

For a **traumatic ET intubation** resulting in soft palate injury, assign code K91.72, Accidental puncture and laceration of a digestive system organ or structure during other procedure. Even if this is documented as "traumatic," traumatic injury codes are not assigned for injuries that occur during or as a result of a medical intervention. See Coding Clinic 2019 Second Quarter p. 23.

For a **laceration** of the right atrial appendage following cardiac pacemaker lead extraction resulting in a pericardial effusion requiring pericardiotomy and suture, assign code I97.51, Accidental puncture and laceration of a circulatory system organ or structure during a circulatory system procedure. See Coding Clinic 2019 Second Quarter p. 24.

A durotomy, or **dural tear**, due to previous epidural injections is assigned to code G96.11, non-traumatic dural tear. Assign code G97.41, Accidental puncture or laceration of dura during a procedure, if a durotomy occurs during a current operation. See Coding Clinic 2014 Fourth Quarter p. 24.

Patient Safety Indicator 15: Abdominopelvic Accidental Puncture or Laceration Rate

All secondary diagnosis codes for accidental puncture or laceration to an organ system except those occurring outside the abdominopelvic region are included in PSI-15. A total of 14 complication codes are included in the measure: D7811-D7812, J9572-J9571, K9171-K9172, E3611-E3612, M96820-M96821, I9751-I9752, N9971-N9972.

Other exceptions include age <18, obstetrical cases, principal diagnosis, and POA = Yes.

PSI-15 is one of 10 PSIs (PSI-90) included in the CMS HAC Reduction Program and only contributes **4%** to the total PSI-90 score.

References

• AHRQ: Patient Safety Indicator 15 (PSI 15) Abdominopelvic Accidental Puncture or Laceration Rate (March 2021).

DEFINITION

The World Health Organization (WHO) defines anemia as a condition in which the number of red blood cells is insufficient to meet the body's physiologic needs.

DIAGNOSTIC CRITERIA

Anemia is measured using the hemoglobin levels:

- Men < 13.0 gm/dl
- Women < 12.0 gm/dl
- Pregnancy < 11.0 gm/dl
- Children > 14 yrs: same as adult
- Children 6 mo–14 yrs < 11.0-12.0 gm/dl depending on age

As a general rule of thumb, one gm/dl of hemoglobin (Hgb) is usually equivalent to a hematocrit (Hct) of 3%. For example, Hgb of 13 gm/dl corresponds to a Hct of 39. A transfusion of 1 unit of blood is expected to increase the Hgb level by about 1 gm/dl.

Acute blood loss anemia is anemia caused by acute bleeding/hemorrhage from any source even if "expected." **Chronic blood loss anemia** is anemia due to chronic blood loss. Causes include gastrointestinal, trauma, surgery, urologic, gynecologic, obstetrical, retroperitoneal.

TREATMENT

Includes monitoring of Hgb/Hct, additional evaluation, frequent vital signs, transfusion, oral or parenteral iron, or rarely erythropoietin.

CODING AND DOCUMENTATION CHALLENGES

The key concept to focus on is "anemia": loss of enough blood to become anemic or more anemic for patients with preexisting chronic anemia. The amount of blood loss is not determinative, only the presence and degree of anemia.

Some patients are chronically anemic and become significantly more anemic with acute bleeding. Anemia may seem intrinsic to or expected with the bleeding that occurred, but is actually an independent measure of severity requiring diagnostic documentation.

No specific criteria have been established for what "significant" is, so providers will have to decide for themselves. Any of the following would suggest a drop in Hgb significant enough to elicit clinical concern:

- Transfusion
- Development of symptoms of anemia not previously present
- Intense serial monitoring of Hgb
- Drop in Hgb of 1.0–2.0 gm/dl (1–2 units of blood). A smaller decrease is more significant with a lower baseline.

> **EXAMPLE** Baseline Hgb of 10 gm/dl with a decrease to 9 gm/dl is not nearly as significant as a drop from baseline of 8 gm/dl to 7 gm/dl.

The terminology to describe acute blood loss anemia (D62) includes:

- Acute blood loss anemia (ABLA)
- Anemia due to acute blood loss
- Acute hemorrhagic anemia
- Acute post-hemorrhagic anemia
- Anemia due to postop blood loss

When both acute and chronic blood loss are present, assign only code D62. Acute blood loss anemia is not classified as a complication of care unless it is specified as postoperative hemorrhage.

Transfusion is not required for diagnosis; monitoring serial Hgb is sufficient.

For **DRG Tips,** see DRG 811, Anemia.

References

- WHO: "Haemoglobin concentrations for the diagnosis of anaemia and assessment of severity"
- Coding Clinic 2014 First Quarter p. 15
- Coding Clinic 2017 Third Quarter, p. 27
- Coding Clinic 2018 Third Quarter p. 21–22
- Coding Clinic 2019 Third Quarter p. 17.

DEFINITION

Sudden reduction of kidney function, usually within a period of hours or days. Causes are classified as:

- Pre-renal: dehydration is the most common cause
- Renal (intrarenal): such as acute tubular necrosis (ATN), glomerulonephritis, acute interstitial nephritis, acute papillary necrosis
- Post-renal: obstruction of ureters or bladder

DIAGNOSTIC CRITERIA

The current consensus-based authoritative criteria for acute kidney injury (AKI) come from the National Kidney Foundation KDIGO conference definition.

KDIGO defines AKI (applicable to both **adult** and **pediatric** patients) as any of the following:

1. Increase in creatinine level to ≥ 1.5x baseline (historical or measured), which is known or presumed to have occurred within the prior 7 days; or
2. Increase in creatinine ≥ 0.3 mg/dl *within 48 hours*; or
3. Urine output < 0.5 ml/kg/hr for 6 hours

These criteria apply to patients with and without **CKD**.

When **baseline creatinine is unknown**, KDIGO advises "The lowest SCr [Creatinine level] obtained during a hospitalization is usually equal to or greater than the baseline. This SCr should be used to diagnose (and stage) AKI."

TREATMENT

IV fluid resuscitation/hydration, serial creatinine levels, evaluation of underlying cause, nephrology consult.

CODING AND DOCUMENTATION CHALLENGES

The terms acute renal/kidney failure and acute kidney injury are synonymous and assigned to code N17.9 which is a CC and often the principal diagnosis. AKI is the authoritative professional acronym for acute kidney injury pursuant to the KDIGO consensus definition.

Guidelines for applying the criteria:

AKI Criterion #1: The **1.5 times baseline** criterion is the most commonly used. A creatinine level from 6 months to as much as a year before may be used as a baseline to identify AKI at the time of admission *if* the patient did not have preexisting CKD or another dramatic change in health since then.

If the patient is admitted for an acute illness and the creatinine is >1.5x the past baseline level, it is "presumed" to have occurred within the prior 7 days, and AKI can be diagnosed. In such circumstances the elevated admission creatinine would also be expected to return to or near the historical baseline further confirming it as acute.

> **EXAMPLE** A previously healthy patient is admitted for nausea, vomiting, diarrhea and dehydration with a creatinine level of 2.0. His creatinine level four months ago was 1.0. It is presumed that the creatinine increased to twice the previous level during this acute illness (within 7 days) confirming AKI. His creatinine returned to 1.2 at discharge making the diagnosis of AKI indisputable.

When the creatinine on admission remains elevated at about the same level during hospitalization, it suggests CKD rather than AKI.

AKI Criterion #2: The **≥ 0.3 within 48 hours** criterion can only be applied prospectively when the creatinine has been measured *within the preceding 48 hours*. It requires two separate measurements within 48 hours showing an increase from the first to the second of ≥ 0.3 mg/dl.

> **EXAMPLE** Patient admitted with creatinine of 1.2 has an increase to 1.6 within 36 hours following cardiac catheterization.

AKI Criterion #3: The **urine output criterion of < 0.5 ml/kg/hr** for 6 hours is based on a patient's weight.

> **EXAMPLE** A 150 lb patient with normal creatinine levels has a total urine output of 180 ccs over 6 hours = 0.44 ml/kg/hr, which meets the urine output criterion for AKI. Calculation: 180cc ÷ 68kg ÷ 6 hrs = 0.44.

AKI on CKD. Patients with CKD are vulnerable to AKI with any physiological stress. AKI criteria are applied the same for patients with CKD.

> **EXAMPLES** Patient with CKD and a stated baseline of 1.8 is admitted with a creatinine of 2.5 which decreases to 1.6 with IV fluids. 1.6 is the true baseline and 2.5 is > 1.5x this level. On the other hand, an admission creatinine of 2.0 (with a prior baseline of 1.0) that remains elevated between 1.7—2.0 does not confirm AKI.

See further case examples that follow on the next two pages.

The diagnosis of AKI depends on what the normal baseline for an individual patient is, not the **reference range** for the lab test (often misunderstood as "normal" range). Reference range is a population-based statistic. It does not indicate what is normal for an individual. AKI creatinine criteria are applied to the baseline without regard to the reference range.

> **EXAMPLES** Baseline = 0.4 mg/dl with increase to 0.8 mg/dl in 36 hrs meets both ≥ 0.3 and 1.5x criteria (0.8 is 2x baseline of 0.4 = a substantial 50% loss of kidney function for this individual).
>
> Creatinine on admission = 1.0 with decrease to 0.5 (baseline) over two days meets 1.5x criterion (1.0 is 2x baseline of 0.5).

BUN should not be used as an indicator of AKI since it can be elevated for many other reasons.

AKI is usually coded first when it is due to dehydration but sequencing is based on the reason for admission.

A **kidney transplant** patient admitted with AKI due to dehydration should be coded to T86.19 (other complication of kidney transplant) with AKI and dehydration as additional diagnoses. The function of the transplanted kidney is affected by the AKI, but the transplant itself has not failed.

73

CASE EXAMPLE 1: AKI CRITERION #1

75-year-old female admitted with severe nausea, vomiting and diarrhea and treated with IV fluids. Unknown baseline.

Creatinine levels admission to discharge: 2.2, 1.6, 1.4, 1.3

This is the most common scenario: a patient is admitted to the hospital with an elevated creatinine, no known baseline, and the creatinine decreases after IV fluids.

Creatinine of 2.2 is 1.7 times higher than the lowest creatinine level of 1.3, and AKI is confirmed based on increase in creatinine to ≥ 1.5 times baseline.

Calculation: 2.2 ÷ 1.3 = 1.7 (Highest ÷ Lowest)

According to KDIGO, when the baseline creatinine is unknown, use the lowest creatinine level measured during admission, which is 1.3 in this case.

CASE EXAMPLE 2: AKI CRITERION #1

62-year-old male admitted with severe nausea, vomiting and diarrhea and treated with IV fluids. Previous creatinine level of 1.1 three months ago.

Creatinine levels admission to discharge: 2.2, 1.6, 1.4, 1.3

This patient's previous creatinine level would be considered his baseline.

Creatinine of 2.2 is 2 times the baseline of 1.1 and AKI is confirmed.

Calculation: 2.2 ÷ 1.1 = 2 (Highest ÷ Baseline)

In this case, the patient's creatinine level returned close to his baseline level of 1.1 at discharge which further confirms AKI.

CASE EXAMPLE 3: AKI CRITERION #2

86-year-old male admitted with heart failure and treated with IV Lasix 80 mg.

Creatinine levels admission to discharge: 0.9, 1.4, 1.1, 0.8

Creatinine increased by 0.5 in 24 hrs (0.9 to 1.4)

Also meets 1.5 times criteria: Calculation: $1.4 \div 0.9 = 1.55$.

CASE EXAMPLE 4: AKI CRITERION #1 - AKI ON CKD

60-year-old with CKD-4 admitted for COVID-19 and pneumonia.

Creatinine admission to discharge: 4.4, 3.0, 2.6, 2.5
GFR admission to discharge: 14, 18, 28, 27

Admission creatinine = 4.4 (1.8 times higher than baseline), which meets the AKI criteria > 1.5 times baseline.

Calculation: $4.4 \div 2.5 = 1.76$

Baseline GFR assumed to be 27 = CKD-4

The five stages of CKD are identified based on the stable baseline GFR.

For *DRG Tips*, see DRGs 682-684, Renal Failure.

References
- KDIGO Clinical Practice Guideline for Acute Kidney Injury. 2012
- Coding Clinic 2019 Second Quarter p. 7.

DEFINITION

Acute tubular necrosis (ATN) is defined as AKI due to an ischemic or toxic injury to and causing dysfunction of the renal tubules which are responsible for fluid and electrolyte regulation. ATN is the cause of AKI in about 30-35% of hospitalized patients.

The distinction between prerenal AKI and ATN is based on the clinical circumstances leading to AKI and the speed of the creatinine response to IV fluid resuscitation.

According to authoritative sources like the National Kidney Foundation and International Society of Nephrology, ATN is a **functional abnormality** of the renal tubules due to toxic or ischemic injury that, if severe, may sometimes progress to necrosis and sloughing of renal tubular cells. Duration of renal tubular dysfunction in ATN ranges from transient dysfunction (> 72 hours) to the prolonged classic picture of pathological tubular necrosis.

The defining feature of ATN is no longer considered to be necrosis as in the past. The term acute tubular injury (ATI) has been proposed but unfortunately did not catch on. Providers are therefore left with the misnomer of acute tubular "necrosis" to describe a condition in which necrosis is usually absent.

Causes of ATN include: IV contrast (always ATN), prolonged hypotension, medications, prolonged pre-renal AKI, rhabdomyolysis with myoglobinuria, tumor necrosis syndrome, chemicals and toxins.

Medications that commonly cause ATN: acetaminophen, NSAIDS, vancomycin, cyclosporine, cisplatin, acyclovir, tetracycline, aminoglycosides.

DIAGNOSTIC CRITERIA

1. Must meet criteria for **AKI.** See *Acute Kidney Injury*.

2. Clinical diagnosis: Expected to take **more than 72 hours** for renal function (measured by creatinine levels) to return near baseline following effective IV fluid resuscitation/hydration.

Other diagnostic lab studies (optional/confirmatory):

- Urine sodium concentration > 40 meq/L (usually < 20 meq/L in prerenal AKI)
- Fractional excretion of sodium (FENa) > 2% but sometimes < 2% (usually < 1% in prerenal AKI).

In the majority of cases the classic urine sediment findings are not present. In fact, the urine sediment may be entirely normal. Urinalysis is no longer used for diagnosis but to exclude other intrarenal conditions like glomerulonephritis and acute interstitial nephritis.

TREATMENT

IV fluid resuscitation/hydration, sometimes combined with IV Lasix if severe; monitoring creatinine levels; correction of offending causes; nephrology consult.

CODING AND DOCUMENTATION CHALLENGES

ATN is commonly under-diagnosed and under-documented creating a frequent query opportunity. Whenever findings suggest that AKI is due to ATN, it should be clarified since ATN is a more specific diagnosis and classified as an MCC.

When documented as "contrast-induced" or due to IV contrast requiring > 72 hours to resolve, it should be clarified as ATN. In cases of AKI following IV contrast where the creatinine returns promptly (within 48 hours or less) to baseline, it is probably not contrast-induced but rather "pre-renal" AKI.

"Vasomotor nephropathy" is a term that is also coded as ATN (N17.0)

References

- KDIGO Clinical Practice Guideline for Acute Kidney Injury. 2012
- UpToDate.com: Pathogenesis, clinical features and diagnosis of contrast-induced nephropathy
- UpToDate.com: Etiology and diagnosis of prerenal disease and acute tubular necrosis in acute kidney injury in adults
- J Am Soc Nephrol 2008 May;19(5):871-875.

DEFINITION

Poisoning is a reaction to the improper use of medication. It includes wrong person, wrong dose, wrong substance, wrong route of administration, combination with alcohol, combination with over-the-counter medications (without MD approval), and overdose.

Adverse effect is a reaction to a medication correctly prescribed and properly administered. Adverse effects include side effects, allergic reaction (hypersensitivity), medication toxicity, reactions caused by interactions between medications, or idiosyncratic (unexpected) reactions.

Underdosing is taking less of a medication than is directed or prescribed or discontinuing use of a prescribed medication on the patient's own initiative. Includes noncompliance and therapeutic error (a complication of care).

Toxic effect is a reaction, consequence, or effect of a *non-medicinal* substance, such as alcohol, animal venom, carbon monoxide, etc.

Drug toxicity due to a medication is not a toxic effect and will be either an adverse effect or poisoning. For example, digoxin toxicity will be an adverse effect if proper use and a poisoning if improper use.

CODING AND DOCUMENTATION CHALLENGES

Poisoning, Adverse Effect, and Underdosing are due to medications, i.e., drugs. Illicit drugs (cocaine, heroin, methamphetamines) are also classified as drugs.

The difference between these three types is use: Poisoning is improper use (wrong drug, overdose, combination with alcohol) and Adverse Effect is proper use (properly taken and administered). Underdosing is improper use but is specifically taking less than prescribed or discontinuing use. Since all are due to drugs, these are classified to the T36-T50 categories.

If the adverse reaction is due to an **illicit drug**, it is always a poisoning since these drugs are never properly taken. An exception is when a condition is due to heavy chronic abuse/dependence which is not considered a poisoning, and a T-code would not be assigned. The condition (manifestation) would be coded first, followed by the code for the drug abuse/dependence (F-code). See Example 4 below.

In some states, marijuana has been legalized for therapeutic and/or recreational use, in others it remains an illicit drug. If legalized for therapeutic use, it would no longer be considered an illicit drug and any adverse reactions could be either a poisoning or adverse effect.

Toxic effects: If the adverse reaction is due to a non-drug (alcohol, venom, bleach ingestion, gas), it is a toxic effect which is listed in the ICD-10 Table of Drugs and Chemicals as "poisoning" but the code description is "toxic effect." The only difference between a poisoning by a drug and "poisoning" by a non-drug (toxin) is the different T code series, T36-T50 for drugs and T51-T65 for non-drugs (toxins).

Poisoning, adverse effects, and underdosing of drugs are classified as T36-T50 (Poisoning by, adverse effects of and underdosing of drugs, medicaments and biological substances). T36–T50 codes identify the (1) Substance, (2) Type: poisoning, adverse effect, or underdosing, (3) Intent (poisoning only), and (4) Encounter: initial, subsequent, or sequela. If the intent is unknown or unspecified, the default is accidental (unintentional).

Toxic effects of non-medicinal substances are classified as T51-T65 (Toxic effects of substances chiefly nonmedicinal as to source) and describe (1) Substance, (2) Intent, and (3) Encounter.

Certain bacterial foodborne intoxications, such as **botulism**, are coded to category A05, not a T-code. In the case of botulism food poisoning (A05.1), the poisoning is due to the clostridium botulinum toxin which is not listed in the table of drugs and chemicals. There are also Excludes1 notes at both A05 and T62 (toxic effect of noxious substances eaten as food). Code A05.1 is specified as "botulism food poisoning" and therefore a more specific code than the T62 codes.

Sequencing. For poisoning and toxic effects, the T-code for the offending substance (drug or non-drug) is sequenced first followed by the manifestations. For adverse effects and underdosing, the manifestation code is sequenced first followed by the code for the type of medication and effect.

The 7th digit for these codes identifies the encounter: initial (A), subsequent (D) and sequela (S). A sequela is a condition or complication that arises later following the initial poisoning, adverse effect, underdosing or toxic effect and is directly related to it.

EXAMPLES STEMI due to recent cocaine use. Cocaine poisoning, accidental, initial episode (T40.5X1A) is the principal diagnosis code followed by STEMI (I21.3).

Erosive esophagitis due to accidental ingestion of bleach. The toxic effect code (T54.91XA) is sequenced first, followed by erosive esophagitis (K22.10).

AKI due to Lasix properly taken and prescribed. AKI (N17.9) is the principal diagnosis followed by adverse effect of loop diuretics (T50.1X5A).

Acute congestive heart failure due to long term methamphetamine abuse with methamphetamine cardiomyopathy. Acute heart failure (I50.9) is the principal diagnosis, with the appropriate code from subcategory F15.1 for the methamphetamine abuse. This would not be classified as a poisoning or adverse effect since the condition is caused by heavy chronic methamphetamine use, not a single dose causing an adverse reaction.

Cannabinoid hyperemesis syndrome is assigned code R11.2, nausea and vomiting, with the appropriate code from category F12, Cannabis related disorders. According to Coding Clinic, poisoning by cannabis is not appropriate since this syndrome is caused by heavy chronic marijuana use, not a single use.

For **DRG Tips**, see DRGs 917-918, Poisoning & toxic effect of drugs.

References

- Official Coding Guidelines Section I.C.19.e
- Coding Clinic 2016 Second Quarter p. 8: Default Intent for Poisoning
- Coding Clinic 2020 First Quarter p. 8: Cannabinoid Hyperemesis Syndrome Associated with Excessive Cannabis Use

DEFINITION

Antimicrobial resistance is resistance of micro-organisms like bacteria, viruses, fungi, and parasites to one or more classes of antimicrobial drugs.

Antibiotic resistance is resistance of bacteria to one or more classes of antibiotics.

Multi-drug resistance (MDR) is resistance of micro-organisms to one or more antibiotics in three or more antibiotic classes.

Antimicrobial resistance is the result of drug overuse and occurs when microorganisms have been exposed to several different drugs over long periods of time.

DIAGNOSTIC CRITERIA

Sensitivity testing demonstrates resistance to one or more drug classes.

Most common drug-resistant organisms encountered among inpatients are: Staphylococcus aureus (MRSA), Enterococcus faecium (potential resistance to all currently used antibiotics), Streptococcus pneumoniae (Pneumococcus), gram-negative coliforms (primarily Klebsiella pneumoniae and E. coli), Pseudomonas, Acinetobacter, Clostridium difficile (C. diff), Candida.

The incidence of MDR tuberculosis infection is rapidly increasing and particularly worrisome because many strains are resistant to all known antitubercular drugs. MDR Candida species are becoming problematic. Many viral pathogens are becoming resistant to multiple drugs.

High-risk MDR circumstances may include: immunosuppression of any cause, indwelling catheters, ventilator status/recently ventilated, recently hospitalized (especially ICU), recent antibiotic therapy (especially broad-spectrum), structural lung disease like bronchiectasis and cystic fibrosis (Pseudomonas), personal history of an MDR infection or known MDR colonization, direct exposure to another person's MDR infection in any setting but especially in home.

Most common situations associated with MDR infections are ventilator associated pneumonia (VAP), catheter-related bloodstream infection (CRBSI), and catheter-associated urinary tract infections (CAUTI).

TREATMENT

Treatment of MDR infections typically requires one or more potent, broad-spectrum antibiotic like vancomycin, gentamicin, piperacillin, cefepime, imipenem/tazobactam often for 14 days or more.

CODING AND DOCUMENTATION CHALLENGES

All category Z16 codes are CCs, hence the important of documentation and coding.

Review the culture sensitivity reports for resistance to even one antibiotic as an opportunity to query for antimicrobial/antibacterial resistance not yet documented by a provider. The provider must document an infection has become drug resistant, e.g., "multi-drug resistant" or "resistant to [specified drug]." If not, a query may be necessary. Do not assign a Z16 category code if the infection identifies the drug resistance, e.g., MRSA pneumonia.

Drug resistance codes (category Z16) identify the antibiotics to which the infectious organism is resistant. Assign codes from category Z16 only when resistance is documented by a provider, not from culture results.

If individual or multiple drugs to which an organism is resistant are documented by the clinician, a code is assigned for each of the drugs identified.

References

- UpToDate.com. Infections and antimicrobial resistance in the intensive care unit: Epidemiology and prevention.
- Drugs.com: www.drugs.com/drug-class.

DEFINITION

Asthma is a chronic inflammatory disorder of the airways characterized by variable and recurring symptoms, airflow obstruction, bronchial hyper-responsiveness (bronchospasm, edema, and hypersecretion). Permanent airway damage may eventually occur leading to COPD (chronic obstructive pulmonary disease).

Predisposition to asthma is genetically determined but clinical asthma also depends on interaction with precipitating environmental factors. Viral respiratory infections are one of the most important causes of asthma exacerbation and may also contribute to the development of asthma in the first place.

Characteristic symptoms of asthma include recurrent episodes of wheezing, dyspnea, chest tightness, and coughing. Asthma may occur alone or in combination with other chronic lung disease (including COPD).

Acute bronchitis is characterized by cough, with or without sputum production, which lasts for at least five days. It is typically self-limited, resolving within one to three weeks. Symptoms result from inflammation of the lower respiratory tract and are most frequently due to viral infection.

COPD is defined as persistent respiratory symptoms and airflow limitation (obstruction) that is not fully reversible due to a combination of obstructive small airway disease and alveolar destruction (emphysema). It typically results from exposure to noxious particles or gases, most commonly tobacco smoke.

Movement of air in and out of the lungs is impaired as is gas exchange (oxygen and carbon dioxide) in the alveoli eventually causing hypoxemia and/or hypercapnia (elevated CO2) commonly progressing to chronic respiratory failure.

Characteristic symptoms of COPD include recurrent episodes of wheezing, dyspnea (shortness of breath) on exertion and/or at rest, coughing and sputum production. COPD may occur alone or in combination with other chronic lung disease such as asthma.

Patients may also have chronic pulmonary heart disease (cor pulmonale) caused by co-existing pulmonary hypertension. See **Pulmonary Heart Disease (Cor Pulmonale).**

Acute exacerbation of COPD (AECOPD) is characterized by acute worsening of symptoms and/or baseline blood gases. Symptoms may include dyspnea, cough, wheezing, sputum production, tachypnea.

Emphysema (permanent over-inflation of the lungs), is caused by destruction of alveoli and damage to small airways (bronchioles), but it is only one component of COPD. Imaging like chest x-ray or CT scan may demonstrate "emphysema" or "hyperinflation."

Chronic obstructive asthma is a term that describes patients who exhibit a combination of COPD and asthma.

Chronic bronchitis is another component (not always present) defined as the presence of cough and sputum production for at least three months in each of two consecutive years. Damage to bronchi (large airways) often results in mucous secretion and bronchospasm especially with acute exacerbations.

DIAGNOSTIC CRITERIA

Asthma. *Intermittent* asthma describes symptoms of wheezing and coughing that occur no more than two days a week. *Persistent* asthma causes symptoms more often than two days a week or two nights per month. There are three levels of severity: mild, moderate, severe.

Acute exacerbation: Acute or subacute episodes of progressively worsening symptoms characterized by decreases (from baseline) in expiratory airflow documented by bedside PEF or with spirometry.

Status asthmaticus: Clinically defined as acute severe asthma (exacerbation) unresponsive to repeated courses of beta-agonist therapy—a minimum of 3 treatments. "Status" means "unchanged."

COPD. Diagnosis is based on a combination of symptoms, imaging and spirometry. Spirometry assesses airflow obstruction and classifies the severity of COPD primarily using the forced expiratory volume in one second (FEV1): mild, moderate, severe, and very severe.

TREATMENT

Chronic: Multiple chronic maintenance and intermittent medications, oral steroids and inhaled nebulizers like albuterol, Atrovent (ipratropium), combination (Combivent), steroids.

Acute: Inhaled beta-agonist bronchodilator (albuterol), steroids (systemic), oxygen and humidification, hydration, supportive care, sometimes inhaled Atrovent if severe. Bedside spirometry (PEF) should always be measured in acute asthma.

Antibiotics are typically administered for AECOPD or bronchitis — less often in acute asthma unless bacterial infection is strongly suspected.

CODING AND DOCUMENTATION CHALLENGES

Asthma as well as asthma and bronchitis associated with COPD are assigned to J44.9 (a non-CC). The documentation that affects DRG assignment is the specification of (acute) exacerbation of COPD or asthma with status asthmaticus, both CCs.

Respiratory failure (MCC) commonly occurs with acute exacerbation in both COPD and asthma and would typically be expected in status asthmaticus. See *Respiratory Failure*.

Assign only code J43.9 Emphysema for an exacerbation of COPD in a patient with emphysema (Excludes 1 note at category J44).

For *DRG Tips*, see DRGs 190-192, COPD, and DRGs 202-203, Bronchitis & asthma.

References

- 2021 Global Initiative for Chronic Lung Disease
  - Chapter 12: Asthma: Principles of Treatment. Allergy Asthma Proc 2012;33 Suppl 1: S47–50.
- NIH: Guidelines for the Diagnosis and Management of Asthma (EPR-3)
- Coding Clinic 2019 First Quarter p. 34-35.

DEFINITION

Body mass index (BMI) is a generally reliable indirect measure of body fat and is calculated by using body weight and height.

Obesity may be classified as **morbid** (BMI ≥ 40) or **severe** (BMI 35.0-39.9) with at least one significant obesity-related comorbidity such as type 2 diabetes, hypertension, sleep apnea, etc. These BMIs for morbid and severity obesity conform with the indications for bariatric surgery.

Obesity hypoventilation syndrome (OHS), also known as Pickwickian syndrome, is a condition in which poor breathing in obese patients results in daytime somnolence with hypoxemia and hypercapnia.

The BMI Table at the end of *Comorbid Conditions* shows BMIs between 19 and 40 for a range of heights and weights. To calculate a BMI, go to an on-line BMI calculator.

DIAGNOSTIC CRITERIA

All patients should have height and weight measured for each admission, or at least a recent reliable measurement.

A BMI of 18.5 to 24.9 is considered normal by the CDC.

BMI	Clinical indicator of
≥ 40.0	Morbid obesity
35–39.9	Severe obesity (with comorbidity)
30–39.9	Obesity
25–29.9	Overweight
< 18.5	Underweight or mild malnutrition
< 17	Moderate malnutrition
< 16	Severe malnutrition

Obesity is also subdivided into three classes: Class 1 (BMI 30 to < 35), Class 2 (BMI 35 to < 40), and Class 3 (BMI ≥ 40).

CODING AND DOCUMENTATION CHALLENGES

Code assignment of BMI can be based on medical record documentation by a non-physician.

BMI cannot be coded unless there is an associated, reportable diagnosis documented by a provider such as obesity of any severity, overweight, OHS, malnutrition, anorexia, underweight, etc.

The diagnosis must meet the definition of an additional diagnosis stated by OCG Section III, Reporting Additional Diagnoses. According to Coding Clinic 2018 Fourth Quarter, p. 77, "Obesity and morbid obesity are **always clinically significant** and reportable when documented by the provider" thereby meeting this requirement.

Patients with substantial edema or ascites, many of whom are malnourished, usually have a BMI somewhat higher than their true "dry-weight" BMI. Highly muscular athletes tend to have falsely high BMI. High-intensity, high-endurance athletes tend to have a clinically insignificant low BMI.

While **Class 3 obesity** is equivalent to morbid obesity, it must be stated as such since ICD-10 does not recognize the obesity classes.

A BMI $\geq$ 40.0 (Z68.4-), BMI < 19.9 (Z68.1) and OHS (E66.2) are CCs.

CMS-HCC 22 includes morbid/severe obesity (E66.01), BMI $\geq$ 40, and OHS.

There are also four pediatric BMI codes (ages 2–20) based on percentile for age: codes Z68.51–Z68.54.

References

- CDC: Defining Adult Overweight and Obesity
- NIH: Managing Overweight and Obesity in Adults
- NIH: Obesity Surgery Indications and Contraindications
- Health Effects of Overweight and Obesity in 195 Countries over 25 Years. N Engl J Med. 2017; 377: 13-27
- Official Coding Guidelines Sections I.C.19.a and I.C.19.c
- Coding Clinic 2018 Fourth Quarter p. 77.

DEFINITION

The sudden cessation of cardiac activity with hemodynamic collapse. In some cases, the heart may have some EKG activity but no discernable cardiac output: pulseless electrical activity (PEA).

Common causes include ventricular fibrillation (most common cause) associated with acute MI, CHF, CAD, hypertensive cardiomyopathy; massive pulmonary embolism; cardiac tamponade; profound hemorrhage (traumatic or non-traumatic), severe electrolyte imbalance; intracranial hemorrhage; medication and drug toxicity; poisons; and some others.

TREATMENT

CPR, defibrillation, epinephrine, treatment of underlying cause.

CODING AND DOCUMENTATION CHALLENGES

The underlying cause is sequenced first. If the cause is unknown, cardiac arrest is used as a principal diagnosis almost exclusively when the patient dies before admission. Usually the principal reason for admission is a consequence of the cardiac arrest.

Do not assign code I46.9 (cardiac arrest) for an EKG finding of **"asystole"** for a brief pause of cardiac activity that terminates spontaneously.

As a secondary diagnosis it is an MCC, but only if the patient survives to discharge. It must be POA to be classified as an SOI-4/ROM-4 diagnosis.

For *DRG Tips*, see DRGs 296-298, Cardiac Arrest, Unexplained.

References

- UpToDate.com: Overview of sudden cardiac arrest and sudden cardiac death
- UpToDate.com: Pathophysiology and etiology of sudden cardiac arrest
- Coding Clinic 2013 First Quarter p. 10
- Coding Clinic 2019 Second Quarter p. 4-5.

DEFINITION

Atrial fibrillation (Afib) represents loss of the regular and organized atrial contraction caused by disordered, chaotic atrial electrical activity with irregular AV-node conduction to the ventricle. It is the most common cardiac arrhythmia. There are four types:

- *Paroxysmal*—Afib which terminates spontaneously or with intervention within 7 days of acute onset.
- *Persistent*—Continuous afib that fails to terminate with treatment to restore sinus rhythm within 7 days of acute onset. Electricocardioversion or pharmacologic therapy intended to restore sinus rhythm.
- *Long-standing persistent*—Persistent afib lasting > 12 months.
- *Permanent*—Treatment with medication for rate control only. No intent to restore sinus rhythm.

Atrial flutter is characterized by a rapid, regular atrial rate about 260-340 typically with 2:1 AV-nodal block where about one-half the atrial beats get through to the ventricles resulting in a regular ventricular rate of about 130-170.

Atrial fib/flutter is a variant of afib with variable, changing EKG patterns of both fibrillation and flutter.

Supraventricular tachycardia (SVT) is an abnormal heart rhythm originating at or above the atrioventricular node and includes atrial, junctional or nodal tachycardia; paroxysmal atrial tachycardia (PAT); and paroxysmal supraventricular atrial tachycardia (PSVT).

Ventricular tachycardia (Vtach) refers to any abnormal ventricular beats > 100 beats/minute, with 3 or more irregular beats in a row. It may be sustained or transient.

Ventricular flutter is a rapid variant of Vtach with no cardiac output (cardiac arrest).

Ventricular fibrillation (Vfib) is an abnormally irregular heart rhythm with no discernable P-, QRS, or T-waves on EKG caused by rapid, uncoordinated fluttering contractions of the ventricles with no cardiac output (cardiac arrest).

Vtach and Vfib occur commonly with acute MI, severe CHF, electrolyte imbalance and certain drug toxicities or poisoning.

Reperfusion ectopy, i.e, tachyarrhythmias such as V-tach or V-fib, commonly occur when blood flow is restored to the heart following interventions to relieve coronary obstruction, such as CABG, PCI, thrombolysis. Reperfusion arrhythmias occur in 80-90% of cases following thrombolytic therapy and PCI and frequently after aortic artery cross clamp release after CABG or other cardiac surgery.

Reperfusion injury is characterized by arrhythmias combined with myocardial ischemia following the above revascularization procedures and is usually a postprocedural complication.

TREATMENT

Atrial fibrillation may be treated with:

- *Rhythm control* (conversion to sinus rhythm) involves electrocardioversion, pharmacological therapy, or catheter ablation. Usually employed with acute paroxysmal afib and when it becomes persistent. Rhythm control may be required immediately (usually by electrocardioversion) especially when hemodynamically unstable. If stable, pharmacologic conversion is typically employed using medications that slow the heart rate (e.g., IV diltiazem or verapamil). Once afib is converted to sinus rhythm, it is usually maintained with amiodarone, dofetilide, flecainide, propafenone, or sotalol to prevent a recurrence.

- *Rate control*: Medication is given to slow the ventricular rate to a normal range without an intent to convert to sinus rhythm. Used for permanent (chronic) afib for long-term treatment and when these patients are admitted with an uncontrolled rate. Beta blockers (like atenolol, metoprolol, carvedilol) are usually used for rate control. Calcium channel blockers (verapamil, diltiazem) may also be used for certain patients. Since the atria continue to fibrillate, anticoagulant therapy is required with the rate control approach to prevent cardiac thrombi and embolism.

Atrial flutter is managed like afib but usually requires prompt conversion since it tends to be more symptomatic and rate control may be more difficult. Catheter ablation is also an effective and definitive therapy.

SVT is managed acutely with IV adenosine or calcium channel blockers like diltiazem (Cardizem). In some cases transient SVT is not treated at all but simply monitored. Long-term treatment may involve calcium channel blockers, digoxin, beta-blockers, or catheter ablation.

Vtach/Vflutter is managed with electrocardioversion and/or anti-arrhythmic medication like lidocaine and others if required.

Vfib is immediately life-threatening and requires emergent CPR and defibrillation.

CODING AND DOCUMENTATION CHALLENGES

Atrial fibrillation specified as chronic (I48.20), permanent (I48.21, persistent (I48.19), and long-standing persistent (I48.11) are CCs. Unspecified (I48.91) and paroxysmal atrial fibrillation (I48.0) are non-CCs.

"**Chronic**" atrial fibrillation (I48.20) is a non-specific term indicating that atrial fibrillation of any type has been present more than three months.

When a patient who has had an acute episode of paroxysmal atrial fibrillation that has been converted to sinus rhythm requiring on-going maintenance medication to prevent occurrences, it represents a chronic condition (if present > 3 months). Likewise, a patient who takes rate control medication with no plans for conversion to sinus rhythm has "**permanent**" atrial fibrillation (I48.21). Query the provider if not specified.

According to Coding Clinic 2018 Third Quarter, a patient admitted with a diagnosis of chronic atrial fibrillation with rapid ventricular response indicates problems with rate control, not paroxysmal atrial fibrillation, and should be coded as chronic atrial fibrillation.

Patients who have had only one episode of paroxysmal afib generally do not require medications for it and would be considered a "history of" afib. Those who have had recurrences that require medication to prevent them would be considered a chronic condition.

Should **multiple types** of afib be documented in the record, such as chronic, persistent afib, only one code should be assigned. Since chronic is non-specific, only persistent afib would be coded. See Coding Clinic 2019 Second Quarter.

It is appropriate to code the specific condition, such as sick sinus syndrome or other significant heart rhythm abnormality, with the **presence of a cardiac device** (pacemaker, AICD, etc.). For example, although sick sinus syndrome is being managed/monitored by a cardiac pacemaker, it would be considered a reportable chronic condition. See Coding Clinic 2019 First Quarter.

Patients who have had a **cardiac ablation** usually no longer have the cardiac arrhythmia. However, if following cardiac ablation for afib the patient still requires medication to prevent recurrences, the patient still has afib.

SVT, PAT, and Vtach characterized by sustained or > 3 beat runs in the progress notes or telemetry strips are typically monitored and do affect inpatient care, if not requiring specific treatment.

SVT and Vtach are CCs. Ventricular flutter is an MCC, and ventricular fibrillation is only an MCC if the patient is discharged alive.

Since **reperfusion ectopy** (arrhythmia) is common and usually transient, do not assign a code for the ventricular arrhythmia unless it is prolonged or causes an injury (e.g., myocardial ischemia) or complication that requires further management and treatment, in which case a complication code should also be assigned if so stated by the provider.

References

- 2014 AHA/ACC/Heart Rhythm Society Guidelines for the Management of Patients With Atrial Fibrillation
- 2015 AHA/ACC/Heart Rhythm Society Guidelines for the Management of Adult Patients With Supraventricular Tachycardia
- Cleveland Clinic Center for Continuing Education: Atrial Fibrillation (August 2018)
- UpToDate.com: Overview of atrial fibrillation
- UpToDate.com: Control of ventricular rate in atrial fibrillation: Pharmacologic therapy
- Merck Manual: Atrial flutter (2017)
- Arrhythmias following Revascularization Procedures in the Course of Acute Myocardial Infarction: Are They Indicators of Reperfusion or Ongoing Ischemia? Scientific World Journal 2013: ID 160380
- Fundamentals of Reperfusion Injury for the Clinical Cardiologist
- Coding Clinic 2018 Third Quarter p. 6
- Coding Clinic 2019 First Quarter p. 33
- Coding Clinic 2019 Second Quarter p. 3-4.

DEFINITION

Cerebral (brain) edema: Swelling/edema within the brain. Common causes: trauma, neoplasm, CVA, intracerebral hemorrhage, anoxic brain injury, post-surgical, brain abscess, encephalitis, toxins, and extreme electrolyte imbalance.

Cerebral (brain) compression: Pressure on the brain due to external (e.g., subdural) or internal (e.g., CVA) mass effect causing displacement and sometimes herniation. Common causes: cerebral edema, traumatic brain injury, any intracranial mass including neoplasm, hemorrhage/hematoma, hydrocephalus, brain abscess.

Cerebral (brain) herniation: Displacement of a part of the brain across/through a fixed intracranial structure such as the falx, tentorium, or foramen magnum that may occur if cerebral edema or compression are severe.

DIAGNOSTIC CRITERIA

Brain CT is usually employed. MRI also clearly demonstrates edema or compression (with or without herniation) but may provide additional information. Cerebral edema is manifested as an area(s) of decreased/low brain density and sometimes described as vasogenic.

Imaging studies in cerebral compression or herniation may show mass effect, midline shift, effacement (appearing inconspicuous or obliterated) of ventricles and/or cerebral sulci (the depressions/grooves of the cerebral cortex between gyri), a "space-occupying lesion" or acute hydrocephalus.

TREATMENT

Treatment of cerebral edema or compression/herniation begins with general supportive measures, control of blood pressure, monitoring of mental status. Other measures may include intracranial pressure monitoring, IV steroids (e.g., decadron), IV diuretics, anticonvulsants, mannitol, hypertonic saline, and others. Surgery may be required for life-threatening herniation.

CODING AND DOCUMENTATION CHALLENGES

Clinical validation of cerebral edema requires clinically significant or generalized brain swelling/edema, not just minor localized edema surrounding a lesion noted on CT or MRI which may be an intrinsic finding associated with the underlying cause especially neoplasms.

Providers sometimes fail to document cerebral compression or herniation when imaging demonstrates mass effect, midline shift, or effacement so a query may be necessary. Cerebral compression or herniation is always clinically significant and may require a query.

Nontraumatic brain compression or **herniation** is captured with code G93.5 (compression of brain). Traumatic brain compression is assigned to new FY2022 codes S06.A1XA and S06.A0XA, Traumatic brain compression with or without herniation. Code also any open wound of head or skull fracture.

Two codes are captured for traumatic brain hemorrhage with cerebral edema: traumatic intracranial hemorrhage (S06.34- or S06.35-) and traumatic cerebral edema (S06.1-). See Coding Clinic 2019 Third Quarter.

Closed head injury (blunt head trauma) may be associated with functional or structural brain or intracranial injury such a hemorrhage, brain contusion, cerebral edema, concussion or loss of consciousness. Make sure than any of these secondary injuries are specifically documented and not simply non-specific "head injury."

Documentation of **GSW [gun shot wound] to the head** is assigned a code for a simple "open wound" or "puncture wound." In most cases, GSWs are associated with life-threatening traumatic hemorrhagic or diffuse intracranial brain injury which should always be specifically documented for correct code and DRG assignment. Look also for skull fracture, brain edema or herniation, GCS component scores and/or "brain death."

For **DRG Tips**, see DRGs 82-84, Traumatic stupor & coma, coma > 1 hour, and DRGs 604-605, Trauma to the skin, subcut tissue & breast.

References

- Cerebral Edema and its Management MJAFI 2003;59: 326-331
- UpToDate.com: Evaluation and management of elevated intracranial pressure in adults
- Cerebral Edema and Its Management: Med J Armed Forces India. 2003; 59: 326-331
- Neuropathology—Chapter 4: Traumatic Brain Injury and Increased Intracranial Pressure
- Radiopaedia.org: Vasogenic cerebral edema
- Coding Clinic 2019 Third Quarter p. 35
- Coding Clinic 2020 Second Quarter p. 31

DEFINITION

Cerebral palsy is a group of non-progressive clinical syndromes characterized by motor and postural dysfunction. Most cases are due to prenatal factors, although perinatal hypoxia-ischemia plays a role in some. Prematurity is commonly associated.

The various types of cerebral palsy include spastic (the most common form), dyskinetic, ataxic, quadriplegia (both arms and legs are affected), diplegia/paraplegia (both legs are affected), hemiplegia (one side of the body is affected).

TREATMENT

The goal of treatment is to help the person be as independent as possible and is directed toward social and emotional development, communication, education, nutrition, mobility, and maximal independence in activities of daily living.

CODING AND DOCUMENTATION CHALLENGES

About 40–65% of children with cerebral palsy have intellectual disability. Documentation should include the degree of weakness or paralysis and the intellectual disability and severity.

Cerebral palsy specified as spastic, athetoid, dyskinetic, dystonic (G80.1, G80.2, G80.3) are CCs. Spastic quadriplegic cerebral palsy (G80.0) is an MCC. Only spastic quadriplegic and athetoid are SOI-2.

All cerebral palsy codes (G80.0 to G80.9) are included in CMS-HCC 74.

References
- UpToDate.com: Cerebral palsy: Overview of management and prognosis
- UpToDate.com: Cerebral palsy: Clinical features and classification.

DEFINITION

Brain infarction or hemorrhage usually associated with permanent or temporary neurologic deficits; includes transient focal neurologic deficits lasting longer than 24 hours.

DIAGNOSTIC CRITERIA

Clinical indicators should be easily identified:

- Positive MRI or CT showing acute infarction or hemorrhage, or
- Persistent focal neurologic defect (> 24 hrs from onset) regardless of imaging

MRI without contrast, if available, is probably the best test to evaluate acute CVA (infarction or hemorrhage); CT is typically used acutely to rule out hemorrhage. Non-hemorrhagic CVA may not be visible on CT during the first 24 hours, only becoming evident after several days.

TREATMENT

- Anti-platelet or anti-thrombotic therapy
- Frequent neurologic assessment (usually every 4–6 hours)
- Evaluation of possible causes: Carotid Doppler, CT scan, MRI, MRA, echocardiogram
- Neurology consult
- TPA (tissue plasminogen activator)

CODING AND DOCUMENTATION CHALLENGES

Some providers may not be aware that a focal neurologic deficit > 24 hours from onset is a stroke (CVA), not a TIA. Duration of neurologic deficit is counted from onset, not presentation. Many patients present to the ER having had several hours or more of symptoms.

The hemorrhage or infarction can be further specified to the affected artery with laterality based on MRI/MRA findings. This specification has no impact on the DRG assignment. Once a CVA has been definitively diagnosed by a provider, coders may assign greater specificity based on other medical record sources such as imaging reports.

NIHSS Stroke Scale (codes in subcategory R29.7-) can be used in conjunction with acute stroke codes (category I63) to identify the patient's neurological status and the severity of the stroke. The stroke scale codes are sequenced after the stroke code(s) and do not have CC or MCC status. Documentation of the NIHSS stroke scale by clinicians other than a provider, such as a nurse, may be used for coding.

A diagnosis of left-sided **weakness** or weakness of one extremity associated with or due to CVA (either acute or residual from a prior CVA) is coded as hemiplegia or monoplegia respectively even if it resolves by the time of discharge for an acute CVA. For an acute CVA, the code for the CVA and the hemiplegia is coded; if residual from a prior CVA, only a code for the hemiplegia is coded.

Hemiplegia codes are CCs; the monoplegia codes are non-CCs.

TPA infusion is assigned code 3E03317. Patients presenting with symptoms of an acute CVA that resolve with TPA or diagnosed with TIA or precerebral occlusion with TPA infusion are assigned to DRGs 61-63, Ischemic Stroke, Precerebral Occlusion or TIA with Thrombolytic Agent.

If TPA infusion is started in another facility within 24 hours of transfer to the current facility, assign code Z92.82 (status post administration of TPA in a different facility within last 24 hours) whether or not the infusion is continued in the receiving facility.

For **DRG Tips**, see DRGs 64-66, Intracranial hemorrhage or infarction.

References

- Guidelines for the Primary Prevention of Stroke: A Statement for Healthcare Professionals From the American Heart Association/American Stroke Association (2014)
- The Lancet 369: 293–298, 2007
- 2021 Guideline for the Prevention of Stroke in Patients With Stroke and Transient Ischemic Attack. Stroke 2021; 52: e364-e467.
- Coding Clinics: 2013 Fourth Quarter p. 124; 2014 First Quarter p. 23; 2015 First Quarter p. 25; and 2017 First Quarter p. 47.

DEFINITION

A persistent and usually progressive, irreversible loss of kidney function. Chronic kidney disease (CKD) is often associated with many common medical conditions including diabetes (most common cause), hypertension, urinary obstruction, autoimmune diseases, recurrent urinary tract infections, and episode(s) of prior AKI.

Certain medications can cause renal damage that may progress to CKD, such as aspirin, acetaminophen (Tylenol), NSAIDs (non-steroidal anti-inflammatory drugs), antibiotics such as gentamicin.

The KDIGO 2012 Clinical Practice Guideline for Chronic Kidney Disease is the authoritative diagnostic and classification standard for CKD. It defines CKD as "abnormalities of kidney structure or function, present for > 3 months, with implications for health." The glomerular filtration rate (GFR) is generally accepted as the best overall index of kidney function.

DIAGNOSTIC CRITERIA

The diagnostic criteria for CKD are **either** of the following present for **> 3 months:** (1) decreased GFR < 60 ml/min, or (2) objective measures of kidney damage including significant persistent albuminuria, urinary sediment abnormalities, electrolyte and other abnormalities due to renal tubular disorders, abnormalities identified on biopsy, structural abnormalities detected by imaging, or history of kidney transplant.

Five stages of CKD are identified based on the **stable baseline GFR**, followed by ESRD which is dialysis-dependent stage 5.

Stage	GFR	Code
1	≥ 90	N18.1
2	60–89	N18.2
3a	45–59	N18.31
3b	30-44	N18.32
4	15–29	N18.4
5	< 15	N18.5
ESRD		N18.6

The diagnosis of CKD stage 1 and 2 requires the presence of one or more of the markers of kidney damage. A GFR ≥ 60 ml/min is not CKD if there are no markers of kidney damage.

Stages 3-5 are based on GFR alone although such patients often also have evidence of these kidney damage markers. The GFR also varies with age, race, and gender. Lab reports of creatinine values should provide the calculated GFR for both African American and non-African American.

CODING AND DOCUMENTATION CHALLENGES

The GFR and therefore the stage of CKD cannot be clinically determined unless or until the GFR/creatinine level is **stable**. Creatinine levels often fluctuate widely during admissions, so great care should be taken in querying for or coding CKD unless there is clear evidence of a stable creatinine level. Even when considered stable, the lowest creatinine level (highest GFR) should be used as the baseline for staging.

Whenever the current creatinine level is lower (higher GFR) than a previously documented level or stage, the current level and stage are the true current baseline but may require clarification if not properly documented.

For example, initial documentation indicates CKD stage 4 with baseline Cr/GFR = 3.0/25. The current lab report shows a stable Cr/GFR = 2.5/35. CKD stage is no longer 4, but rather stage 3b. There's no such thing as "double" stage CKD like stage 3/4, and the lowest stage (highest GFR) should always be used.

Ideally for accurate data collection, the stage should be specified in all cases of CKD. Stages 4 and 5 are CCs. Stages 1 to 3 are not CCs, but stage 3 is CMS-HCC 138 (version 24.0). Stage 3 is assigned code N18.31 for stage 3A, N18.32 for stage 3B, and N18.30 if unspecified.

Chronic renal insufficiency, chronic renal failure, or chronic renal disease may be used as equivalent terms for CKD but should be staged.

A patient with chronic kidney disease requiring chronic dialysis is coded as N18.6, End stage renal disease. Code Z99.2, Dependence on renal dialysis, should also be coded.

ESRD and transplant status. Clinically, renal transplant patients are still considered to have ESRD which may be documented as such, but for coding purposes if they are not dialysis-dependent, ESRD (N18.6) should not be coded. The current CKD stage is coded along with kidney transplant status (Z94.0).

All kidney transplant patients have CKD based on the CKD diagnostic criteria, but the presence of CKD alone does not constitute a transplant complication.

References

- KDIGO 2012 Clinical Practice Guideline for the Evaluation and Management of Chronic Kidney Disease Kidney International Supplements 2013; 3: 19–62
- Official Coding Guidelines I.C.14.a.2.

DEFINITION

Clostridium difficile, also known as Clostridioides difficile, (C. diff) is a bacterium that produces a toxin that damages the colon. C. diff does not actually cause invasive infection.

Symptoms include severe diarrhea (sometimes hemorrhagic), cramping abdominal pain, fever, and leukocytosis. Can progress rapidly to sepsis. Complications may also include ileus, megacolon, perforation.

Approximately 90-95% of C. diff infections are antibiotic-induced. Symptoms of C. diff can begin during or up to one month after antibiotic therapy, although most cases occur within two weeks of antibiotic therapy. It is highly contagious.

Recurrent C. diff colitis is defined as complete relief of symptoms of initial infection followed by recurrence in 2-8 weeks after treatment stopped. Occurs in up to 25% of patients with C. diff; sometimes multiple episodes.

DIAGNOSTIC CRITERIA

The onset of symptoms, especially related to antibiotic therapy, typically prompts the provider to order a stool test for the toxin or its gene. Cultures are not usually done. A positive test confirms the diagnosis, but it is not 100% accurate so some patients with C. diff might have a negative test and may be treated presumptively for suspected C. diff especially if clinical circumstances are highly suggestive.

TREATMENT

- Cessation of offending antibiotic, IV fluids, oral probiotics, contact precautions
- Oral metronidazole (Flagyl), Fidaxomicin (Dificid), vancomycin, or bezlotoxumab (Zinplava)
- Fecal transplant (bacteriotherapy)

CODING AND DOCUMENTATION CHALLENGES

Occasionally, the provider may decide that C. diff is highly likely based on clinical circumstances when the stool test is **negative**. Documentation should include acknowledgment that the test is negative but C. diff is considered likely on clinical grounds. A full course of therapy would be expected — 10-14 days for antibiotics, one dose for bezlotoxumab.

C. diff infection (colitis/enterocolitis) either initial (A047.2) or recurrent (A047.1) is a CC. A diagnosis of "pseudomembranous colitis" is coded as C. diff.

For **DRG Tips**, see DRGs 371–373, Major GI disorders & peritoneal infections.

References
- UpToDate.com: Clostridioides difficile infection in adults: Clinical manifestations and diagnosis
- UpToDate.com: Clostridioides difficile infection in adults: Treatment and prevention
- Clinical Practice Guidelines for Clostridium difficile Infection in Adults and Children: 2017 Update by the Infectious Diseases Society of America (IDSA) and Society for Healthcare Epidemiology of America (SHEA).

DEFINITION

Coagulation disorders (coagulopathies) are disruptions in the body's ability to control blood clotting. Coagulation disorders are either inherited or acquired (e.g., drug-induced or due to liver disease). Inherited coagulation disorders are rare and include hemophilia, von Willebrand disease, factor XI deficiency, and fibrinogen disorders.

Acquired coagulation disorders commonly occur and are the focus of this section. Common causes of acquired coagulation disorders are those due to anticoagulant/antithrombotic therapy or liver disease.

Anticoagulants interfere with normal clotting factors (e.g., prothrombin, thrombin, Factor X). Antithrombotics interfere with platelet function that is also necessary for proper clot formation.

Anticoagulant medications include Coumadin, heparin, Lovenox, Factor Xa inhibitors like Eliquis and Xarelto and direct thrombin inhibitors like Pradaxa, Angiomax, Argatroban, Iprivask, and Refludan.

Antithrombotic medications include aspirin ("ASA"), Plavix, Ticlid, Integrilin, Aggrastat, ReoPro, and others.

Patients with acute and chronic **liver disease** often have associated coagulation disorders since the liver produces clotting factors. Severe liver failure results in a deficiency of these factors causing an acquired coagulation disorder.

DIAGNOSTIC CRITERIA

Recognition of acquired coagulation disorders can be a complex process, but bleeding is the principal clinical hallmark.

Anticoagulant drugs act by prolonging the prothrombin time (PT) usually reported as INR (international normalized ratio) and/or aPTT (activated PTT) also commonly called PTT, so elevated INR and/or aPTT would be expected as a therapeutic effect. Severe liver failure also causes elevation of both INR and PTT above the reference range.

An elevated INR or aPTT would be expected as a therapeutic effect, not an adverse effect or toxicity, of these anticoagulants. Similarly elevated INR and aPTT do not represent complications of severe chronic liver disease.

Depending on clinical circumstances the expected therapeutic range for INR is 2.0-3.0 and for aPTT is 1.5-2.5 x the upper limit of reference ("normal") range. Higher levels indicate significant bleeding risks and require medication adjustments. An INR of ≤ 1.1 would be considered normal in healthy individuals.

Antithrombotics interfere with platelet function causing a prolonged bleeding time test. In addition to bleeding, thrombocytopenia is a common complication of antithrombotics.

TREATMENT

Discontinuation of drug, monitoring INR and/or PTT, and/or reversal of the drug effect, e.g., Vitamin K (phytonadione), IV clotting factor replacement, protamine sulfate can be used to reverse the effects of heparin.

CODING AND DOCUMENTATION CHALLENGES

When a patient is admitted with bleeding associated with anticoagulant/antithrombotic therapy, code D68.32 (hemorrhagic disorder due to extrinsic circulating anticoagulants) is assigned. An additional code is used for the site of bleeding.

The **sequencing** of code D68.32 and codes for the type/site of bleeding as principal diagnosis depends on the circumstances of admission. Consider whether the "focus" of the admission was the bleeding itself (e.g., evaluation, procedures, transfusion, monitoring, hemoglobin/hematocrit) or the correction of the bleeding disorder. In either of these situations, an additional code for adverse effect, if applicable, would also be used to identify the drug (T45.515- or T45.525-).

A patient admitted with a bleeding caused by an anticoagulant/antithrombotic drug taken improperly (poisoning), would be assigned to code T45.511- or T45.521- which is assigned as principal diagnosis. Code D68.32 would be assigned as a secondary diagnosis.

Coagulation disorder due to acute or chronic **liver disease** is assigned code D68.4. Coagulation disorder due to aspirin is coded under subcategory T39.01 (poisoning or adverse effect).

Abnormal PT (INR) or PTT due to an anticoagulant that does not cause bleeding or some other complication is assigned symptom code R79.1, Abnormal coagulation profile.

Likewise, a diagnosis of "**coagulopathy** due to chronic anticoagulation" would be assigned code R79.01, Long term use of anticoagulants, not D68.9, Coagulation defect unspecified, unless there was evidence of bleeding or other complication and would then be assigned to a more specific code or other specified coagulation defect.

> **EXAMPLES** Patient with GI bleeding while properly taking Plavix requiring discontinuation of Plavix, blood transfusion, EGD and colonoscopy and identified as bleeding gastric ulcer. Assign codes K25.4 (gastric ulcer with bleeding) as principal diagnosis with D68.32 (hemorrhagic disorder due to circulating anticoagulants) and T45.525A (adverse effective of antithrombotic) as secondary diagnoses. The ulcer with bleeding was the focus of the admission and an adverse effect of Plavix (antithrombotic).
>
> Patient with epistaxis and taking Coumadin as prescribed is treated with nasal packing and requires admission for fresh frozen plasma to reverse elevated INR of 6.8, discontinuation of Coumadin, serial hemoglobin and INR, and subsequent cautious resumption of Coumadin based on INR. Assign code D68.32 (hemorrhagic disorder due to circulating anticoagulants) as principal diagnosis, with T45.515A (adverse effect of anticoagulants) and R04.0 (epistaxis) as secondary diagnoses.

An **acquired hypercoagulable state** is an increased risk for thrombosis due to clinical conditions such as malignancy, diabetes, pregnancy, postoperative state, myeloproliferative disorders. According to Coding Clinic 2021 Q2, "Patients with atrial fibrillation on chronic anticoagulant therapy may have an increased incidence of acquired hypercoagulable state." If specifically documented by the provider as a "secondary" or "acquired" hypercoagulable state, assign code D68.69, other thrombophilia (a CC). The provider does not have to link the secondary hypercoagulable state to the atrial fibrillation.

References

- UpToDate.com: Direct Oral Anticoagulants (DOACs) and Parenteral Direct Thrombin Inhibitors: Dosing and Adverse Effects
- Coding Clinic 2016 First Quarter p. 14-15
- Official Guidelines for Coding and Reporting Section I.C.19.e.5
- Pesarini, G et al. Current Antithrombotic Therapy in Patients with Acute Coronary Syndrome Undergoing Percutaneous Coronary Interventions: Interventional Cardiology Review 2014; 9: 94-101
- Coding Clinic 2021 Second Quarter p. 8.

DEFINITION

A profound alteration of consciousness (arousal and responsiveness) ranging from obtundation with impaired responsiveness, to unconsciousness with some responsiveness, to complete unresponsiveness.

Typical causes include head trauma, brain (cerebral) edema or compression, CVA/brain hemorrhage (especially brain stem), severe metabolic/physiologic disturbances (e.g., anoxia, hypothermia, many others), organ failure (e.g., hepatic or uremic coma), encephalitis/meningitis, and medications, drugs, and toxins.

Persistent vegetative state is prolonged deep coma.

DIAGNOSTIC CRITERIA

The Glasgow Coma Scale (GCS) is used to objectively describe the extent of impaired consciousness in acute medical and trauma patients. It is based on the patient's best response in three areas: Eye opening (score 1-4), Verbal response (score 1-5), and Motor response (score 1-6).

The lowest possible total GCS is 3 (deep coma or brain death), while the highest is 15 (fully awake person).

- 3–8 points = Severe: Coma
- 9–12 points = Moderate: Stupor/obtundation
- 13–15 points = Minor: Lethargy

Since patients who are intubated are unable to speak, their verbal score cannot be assessed.

GCS criteria for infants and children differ from those for adults.

TREATMENT

Correction of underlying cause; neurologic evaluation and testing, supportive care, and if severe, mechanical ventilation.

CODING AND DOCUMENTATION CHALLENGES

OCG I.C.18.e. no longer allows GCS coding with non-trauma conditions: "The coma scale codes (R40.21- to R40.24-) can be used in conjunction with **traumatic brain injury** codes. These codes are primarily for use by trauma registries, but they may be used in any setting where this information is collected."

The terms "coma" and "unconsciousness" are coded R40.20 which is an MCC. Persistent vegetative state, R40.3, is a CC.

Although the term "**unconsciousness**" is classified as coma, it needs to be a clinically valid diagnosis representing a persistent (not transient) state of altered level of consciousness. Brief loss of consciousness may be nothing more than a symptom intrinsic to some relatively minor condition such as a seizure or syncope, and if so, not coded.

Certain diagnoses are a combination code "with coma" such as hepatic failure or DKA. Review the patient's signs and symptoms and the GCS (total score 3-8 points) to determine whether or not the patient meets the indicators for coma.

A GCS score is usually documented as E+V+M. For example, a GCS E2/V1/M2 (total score = 5) would indicate coma.

The GCS is one of the SOFA score diagnostic criteria for Sepsis-3. A GCS total score of 13-14 equals one point on the SOFA scale.

Codes for coma or GCS scores should not be reported for a patient with a **medically-induced** coma or is sedated.

References

- UpToDate.com: Stupor and Coma in Adults
- CDC: Glasgow Coma Scale
- NIH National Center for Biotechnology Information: Pediatric Version of the Glasgow Coma Scale
- Essentials of Clinical Neurology: Neurology History and Examination, Chapter 9: Stupor and Coma
- Glasgow Coma Scale - Brain Injury Alliance of Utah.

DEFINITION

The 2019 coronavirus infectious disease (COVID-19) is the collective term for all respiratory infections caused by SARS-CoV-2 virus. The Delta variant of SARS-CoV-2 is more readily transmitted than the original Alpha strain and is associated with a higher risk of hospitalization.

Symptoms include fever and/or respiratory-like symptoms such as cough, sneezing, shortness of breath and difficulty breathing. May progress to pneumonia, acute respiratory failure, severe sepsis, acute kidney injury and death.

Direct human contact is the primary mechanism of transmission. The CDC now says that transmission through contact with contaminated surfaces is rare, but possible. Surface sanitation is still recommended.

Risk factors include age 65 or older, obesity, and anyone with serious underlying medical conditions especially those who are immunocompromised.

DIAGNOSTIC CRITERIA

- Positive COVID-19 test result, or
- Definitive documentation of COVID-19 by a provider.

TREATMENT

The best treatment is prevention with vaccination. Treatment of infection is primarily supportive focusing on the complications. Specific treatment modalities for severely ill patients include:

- High-dose steroids (Dexamethasone)
- Remdesivir (antiviral)
- Antibodies: convalescent plasma from individuals who have recovered from COVID-19
- Tocilizumab (Interleukin-6 receptor blocker) + Dexamethasone
- Baricitinib (immunomodulator)

CODING AND DOCUMENTATION CHALLENGES

The ICD-10-CM code for COVID-19 is U07.1. Only confirmed cases of COVID-19 are coded U07.1, defined by a positive COVID-19 test result or provider documentation that the individual has COVID-19. This applies to adult, pediatric and newborn patients.

A positive test result or documentation of the test result in the record is not required when the provider has definitively documented COVID-19. The provider's diagnostic statement that the patient has COVID-19 is sufficient.

When COVID-19 is definitively diagnosed before test results are available and later the test results are negative, a query for clarification is in order to allow the provider to reconsider and reaffirm the diagnosis or document disagreement with a negative test. It is recommended that claims for inpatient admissions or outpatient encounters not be submitted until the COVID-19 test results are available.

Likewise, if based on the clinical indicators the clinical validity of a COVID-19 diagnosis is questionable, query the provider.

Sequencing COVID-19 as principal diagnosis. When COVID-19 meets the definition of principal diagnosis, code U07.1 is assigned first followed by the appropriate codes for the associated manifestations — except when another guideline requires that certain diagnoses be sequenced first, such as sepsis, obstetrics, or transplant complications.

For example, the principal diagnosis for a patient presenting with **sepsis** due to COVID-19 (A41.89 or U07.1) depends on the circumstances of the admission and whether or not sepsis meets the definition of the principal diagnosis. If a patient is admitted with sepsis due to COVID-19 pneumonia and the sepsis meets the definition of principal diagnosis, then viral sepsis (A41.89) should be assigned as principal diagnosis, followed by the codes U07.1 and J12.82.

When the reason for the admission is a respiratory manifestation of COVID-19, assign code U07.1 as the principal diagnosis and assign codes for the respiratory manifestations as secondary diagnoses.

Providers do not have to explicitly link the respiratory condition with COVID-19 since COVID-19 is a respiratory disease caused by SARS-CoV-2. For example:

- **Pneumonia**: For pneumonia due to COVID-19, assign U07.1, COVID-19, and J12.89, Other viral pneumonia.
- **Lower respiratory infection:** U07.1, COVID-19, and J22, Unspecified acute lower respiratory infection
- **Acute respiratory failure or acute respiratory distress syndrome (ARDS)**: U07.1, COVID-19, and J96.00 or J80 (ARDS).

When the reason for the admission is a *non-respiratory* manifestation (e.g., viral enteritis) of COVID-19, assign code U07.1, COVID-19, as the principal diagnosis and assign the code(s) for the manifestation(s) as additional diagnoses. Providers do have to link the non-respiratory condition to COVID-19.

COVID-19 readmissions. The principal diagnosis is dependent on whether the COVID-19 infection has resolved which is determined by provider documentation. If a patient is admitted with a residual effect (sequelae) and the provider documentation indicates the COVID-19 infection *has resolved* or the patient is *no longer infectious* (even with a current or recent positive COVID-19 test), assign a code for the residual effect as principal diagnosis and U09.9, Post-COVID-19 condition. If the COVID-19 infection has *not resolved*, assign code U07.1 as principal diagnosis and the manifestation as a secondary diagnosis.

Other indicators of a "resolved" COVID infection: (1) Greater than 14 days since onset of symptoms or date of positive test, (2) patient not in isolation, (3) lack of COVID-19 treatment (remdesivir, decadron, etc.).

Post COVID-19 condition, new code U09.9, has been added to permit the establishment of a link between a prior COVID-19 and a post-acute sequela. Code U09.9 is not to be used as a principal diagnosis or in cases that are still presenting with active COVID-19. However, an exception is made in cases of re-infection with COVID-19, occurring together with a condition related to prior COVID-19.

Uncertain diagnosis. Do not assign code U07.1 for provider documentation of possible, probable, suspected, or inconclusive COVID-19 or using other terms of uncertainty, as a diagnosis. Instead assign a code(s) explaining the reason for encounter (such as fever) or Z20.828 Contact with and (suspected) exposure to other viral communicable diseases. If the test results come back positive after discharge, code as confirmed COVID-19.

Code Z86.16, **Personal history of COVID-19**, is assigned for a patient who previously had COVID-19 but no longer has COVID-19 or sequelae. Personal history codes explain a patient's past medical condition that no longer exists and not receiving any treatment but may have potential for reoccurrence.

For COVID-19 infections presenting during **pregnancy, childbirth and the puerperium**, assign a code from O98.5-, Other viral diseases complicating pregnancy, childbirth and the puerperium, followed by U07.1 and the pertinent code for the associated infection.

Cytokine release syndrome (CRS), also called cytokine storm, is an acute systemic inflammatory syndrome associated with COVID-19, T-cell therapy, other immunotherapy, allogeneic transplantation, and can be a reaction to certain antibiotics. The underlying cause of CRS is sequenced first, and the manifestation (CRS) as a secondary diagnosis. If a patient is admitted with CRS due to a previous COVID-19 infection and the patient no longer has COVID-19 (which was the underlying cause), the best option at this time without further guidance would be to assign CRS as the principal diagnosis with U09.9, Post-COVID-19 condition. CRS grades 3 to 5 are CCs (codes D89.833-D89.835).

Reference

- UpToDate.com: COVID-19: Management in hospitalized adults
UpToDate.com: Cytokine release syndrome (CRS)
- Official Coding Guidelines Section I.C.1.g.(1): Coronavirus infections

- UpToDate.com: Coronavirus disease 2019 (COVID-19)
- CDC: Coronavirus (COVID-19)
- Coding Clinic 2020 Second Quarter p. 9-1
- Coding Clinic 2021 Fourth Quarter p. 101-10

DEFINITION

Cystic fibrosis (CF) is a hereditary disorder characterized by thick secretions in the lungs, pancreas, liver, intestine, and other organs resulting in multi-system disease. Median survival is about 37 years.

DIAGNOSTIC CRITERIA

- Clinical involvement in one or more organ systems, usually multiple (not required for screened newborns), and
- Elevated sweat chloride (> 60 mmol/L) × 2

About 2% have organ system involvement but non-diagnostic sweat chloride requiring DNA analysis for confirmation. Pulmonary involvement occurs in 90% of patients who survive the neonatal period, and end stage lung disease is the principal cause of death.

Commonly associated organ system complications of CF include:
- **Pulmonary:** Bronchiectasis, sinusitis, bronchitis, recurrent pneumonia, pneumothorax, allergic bronchopulmonary aspergillosis (ABPA), COPD. Patients often have respiratory colonization by bacteria or fungi especially Pseudomonas, Staph, Hemophilus.
- **Gastrointestinal:** Meconium ileus (neonates/infants), intestinal obstruction, failure to thrive, GERD, GI bleeding, biliary cirrhosis, cholelithiasis, liver disease, distal intestinal obstruction syndrome (DIOS), small intestine bacterial overgrowth (SIBO).
- **Pancreatic:** Pancreatic insufficiency with malabsorption and secondary insulin-dependent "CF-related" diabetes, pancreatitis.

TREATMENT

Treatment directed at organ involvement especially:

- Chronic antibiotics (especially azithromycin)
- Bronchodilator therapy; inhaled Pulmozyme—liquefies sputum
- Hypertonic saline nebulizer
- Pancreatic enzyme replacement therapy (PERT)

- Insulin for CF-related diabetes (CFRD)
- GERD: Omeprazole, Tagamet, Pepcid
- Ivacaftor restores deficient CF-protein function for CF patients who have certain specific CF genotypes—about 4% of CF patients

CODING AND DOCUMENTATION CHALLENGES

ICD-10 codes for cystic fibrosis are assigned based on the chronic manifestations affecting the patient to identify which organ systems are involved.

CF unspecified (E84.9) and other specified codes (intestinal, fecal impaction, DIOS, other) are CCs and SOI 2. CF with pulmonary manifestations (E84.0) and with meconium ileus (E84.11) are MCCs and default SOI 3.

Assign multiple CF codes as needed to describe all of the patient's baseline organ involvement. Most patients will have pulmonary involvement plus others.

If a patient is admitted due to a **manifestation** or complication of the CF (such as acute bronchitis, pneumonia, bowel obstruction, pancreatitis, etc.), assign the manifestation or complication as the principal diagnosis, and the CF as a secondary diagnosis.

When the focus of the admission is CF itself rather than a complication or manifestation, CF would be assigned as the principal diagnosis.

References

- UpToDate.com: Cystic fibrosis: Clinical manifestations and diagnosis
- UpToDate.com: Cystic fibrosis: Overview of the treatment of lung disease
- UpToDate.com: Cystic fibrosis: Overview of gastrointestinal disease
- Cystic Fibrosis Foundation (cff.org)
- Coding Clinic 2002 Fourth Quarter p. 45-46.

DEFINITION

Deep vein thrombosis (DVT) describes venous thrombosis in deep veins. Lower extremity DVT (iliac, femoral, popliteal, tibial) is by far the most common but vena cava, subclavian, axillary, renal DVT are not uncommon.

Lower extremity DVT is most notably caused by immobilization, especially in the inpatient setting. Symptoms include warmth, edema, pain and tenderness. Other causes include post-operative, casting of extremity, obesity, oral contraceptives, hormone replacement therapy, pregnancy or postpartum status, hypercoagulable states (hereditary or acquired), and prolonged sitting position (e.g., travel).

There are two main classifications of DVT based on how long the blood clot is present. **Acute DVT** is defined by the presence of a thrombus for ≤ 14 days. **Chronic DVT** occurs when one or more recurrent acute episodes have occurred.

DIAGNOSTIC CRITERIA

Include D-dimer level > 500 ng/mL and positive ultrasound.

TREATMENT

- **Acute DVT** is usually treated with heparin-type medications for immediate anticoagulation to prevent further clot growth. None of these medications actually "treat" the acute DVT. The acute blood clots in deep veins are usually dissolved spontaneously by endogenous processes in the veins within a few days, not by heparin, Coumadin, or Xarelto. A transition is then made to intermediate-term (3-12 months) Coumadin, or more recently Xarelto, to prevent recurrent DVT.

- **Chronic DVT** usually requires chronic life-long anticoagulation (e.g., Coumadin, Xarelto) after the first recurrent episode, and also after the initial episode for patients with certain underlying clotting disorders.

CODING AND DOCUMENTATION CHALLENGES

The acute episode of DVT ends when the patient is stabilized, transitioned to Coumadin or Xarelto and discharged. If such a patient is admitted with a "history of DVT" and without a recurrent episode of DVT, the correct status is "history of DVT," not acute or chronic DVT. A subsequent episode of DVT requiring admission would constitute a recurrent episode of acute DVT.

When recurrent episodes of DVT become "chronic" is a subjective decision requiring physician determination. Factors to be considered are the number and frequency of episodes, and the need for life-long anticoagulant therapy. Long-term (> 1 year) Coumadin or Xarelto for DVT is indicative of chronic DVT, as is the presence of a Greenfield (IVC) filter.

While deep venous phlebitis commonly causes DVT, the term DVT implies that phlebitis (venous inflammation) is absent from both a clinical and coding perspective. The term "thrombophlebitis" indicates the presence of both DVT and phlebitis.

Acute and chronic DVTs are CCs. CMS-HCC 108 includes almost all codes for both acute and chronic thrombosis and thrombophlebitis.

References

- UpToDate.com: Overview of the treatment of lower extremity deep vein thrombosis (DVT)
- UpToDate.com: Clinical presentation and diagnosis of the nonpregnant adult with suspected deep vein thrombosis of the lower extremity
- UpToDate.com: Primary (spontaneous) upper extremity deep vein thrombosis
- American College of Cardiology: Diagnosis and Management of Acute Deep Vein Thrombosis.

DEFINITION

The Diagnostic and Statistical Manual of Mental Disorders version 5 (DSM-5) is the authoritative source for mental disorders.

Major depressive disorder (MDD) is defined as a depressed mood or a loss of interest or pleasure in daily activities including characteristic symptoms nearly every day for more than two weeks with impaired function. To establish a diagnosis of MDD, there must also never have been a manic or hypomanic episode.

Bipolar disorder is also known as manic-depressive illness. Bipolar I represents the modern understanding of manic-depressive illness characterized by severe depression alternating with at least one episode of mania. Bipolar II is characterized as recurring episodes of MDD and at least one hypomanic episode, not full mania.

DIAGNOSTIC CRITERIA

An **MDD episode** is defined by the presence of **all** of the following three criteria (A–C):

A. Cardinal symptoms: **5 or more** of the following (one must be #1 or #2) present during the same two-week period that represents a change from baseline function:

1. Depressed mood most of the day, nearly every day

2. Loss of interest or pleasure in all, or almost all, activities most of the day, nearly every day

3. Weight loss or gain +/− 5% body weight in 1 month (unintentional), or decreased or increased appetite nearly every day

4. Insomnia or hypersomnia nearly every day

5. Psychomotor agitation or retardation nearly every day

6. Fatigue or loss of energy nearly every day

7. Feelings of worthlessness or excessive, inappropriate guilt nearly every day

8. Diminished ability to concentrate ("think") or indecisiveness, nearly every day

    9. Recurrent thoughts (not just fear) of death or recurrent suicidal thoughts, plans, or attempts

B. Symptoms cause clinically significant distress or impairment in social, occupational, or other important areas of functioning.

C. Episode is not attributable to the effects of substance abuse, a psychosis like schizophrenia, or another underlying medical condition

Bipolar I includes both the MDD criteria, and a manic episode: distinct period of persistently elevated, expansive, irritable mood causing marked impairment of social/occupational function, or necessitating hospitalization, or with psychotic features.

Bipolar II is the same as Bipolar I except only hypomanic episode with an uncharacteristic change in function without needing hospitalization or psychotic features.

Remission: **Full** — no significant signs or symptoms for > 2 months following an MDD episode. **Partial** — symptoms of the MDD episode persist but full criteria no longer met, or a period of < 2 months without significant symptoms following an episode.

Episode: **Single** — first occurrence of an MDD episode followed by at least two consecutive months of partial or full remission. **Recurrent** — any subsequent episode of MDD.

Severity:
- **Mild**—a few symptoms, intensity distressing but manageable, minor functional impairment
- **Moderate**—symptoms intermediate between mild and severe
- **Severe**—large number of symptoms, especially suicidal symptoms or deeply withdrawn, intense and unmanageable symptoms, marked functional impairment
- **Psychotic features**—delusions and/or hallucinations

Most patients with depressive symptoms lasting longer than two years will meet MDD criteria during that time, in which case MDD should be the diagnosis.

TREATMENT

Includes psych consult, psychotherapy. Common MDD drugs include Prozac (paroxetine), Buspar. Bipolar disorder drugs include antidepressants (Seroquel, Latuda, Zyrexa, Prozac, Lamictal, Dapakote, Lithium), and anti-mania drugs like Tegretal, Riperdol, Abilify. Electroconvulsive therapy (ECT) is particularly effective in the elderly.

CODING AND DOCUMENTATION CHALLENGES

The greatest challenge for providers is clearly defining and correctly diagnosing major depressive disorder (MDD) and specific types of bipolar disorders in contrast to simply unspecified depression (new code F32.A), MDD (F32.9) or bipolar disorder (F31.9).

Depressive disorder or simply "depression" has symptoms characteristic of MDD or other depressive disorders but does not meet diagnostic criteria or insufficient information to establish the diagnosis.

For the most part, MDD must be specified as single episode or recurrent *and* mild, moderate, or severe to be a CC. However, MDD recurrent (F33.9) or recurrent in remission (F33.40) are also CCs.

Bipolar disorder must be specified as current episode (hypomanic, manic, or depressed) and mild, moderate, or severe to be a CC. Bipolar II disorder and recurrent manic episodes are also CCs.

CMS-HCC 59 includes the above codes, except unspecified depression and MDD.

References

- American Psychiatric Association. Diagnostic and Statistical Manual of Mental Disorders (DSM-5)
- UpToDate.com: Unipolar major depression in adults: choosing initial treatment
- UpToDate.com: Diagnosis and management of late-life unipolar depression
- UpToDate.com: Unipolar depression in adults: treatment of resistant depression
- UpToDate.com: Tricyclic and tetracyclic drugs: pharmacology, administration, and side effects
- UpToDate.com: Unipolar depression in adults: assessment and diagnosis
- UpToDate.com: Bipolar major depression in adults: choosing treatment
- UpToDate.com: Bipolar disorder in adults: clinical features.

DEFINITION

Diabetes mellitus (DM). Disordered glucose regulation due to inadequate insulin production or abnormal cellular resistance to the effects of insulin. DM has primary (type 1 and type 2) causes and secondary causes such as another underlying disease process (e.g., chronic pancreatitis, cystic fibrosis, hemochromatosis) or drugs (e.g., steroids) and toxins (e.g., dioxins used in pesticides).

Common chronic diabetic complications include:

Circulatory: Peripheral vascular/arterial disease (PVD) includes peripheral arteries only, usually lower extremities, diabetic microangiopathy.

Neuropathy: Mono-, poly-, autonomic neuropathy (e.g., gastroparesis), and amyotrophy.

Nephropathy: Chronic kidney disease, glomeruloscleroses.

Retinopathy (opthalmic): Proliferative, non-proliferative, macular edema, or unspecified; diabetic glaucoma is caused by retinopathy. Diabetic cataract, a common and major cause of visual impairment in diabetics, is also an opthalmic complication but unrelated to retinopathy.

Skin: Non-pressure foot ulcer and ischemic and non-ischemic non-pressure ulcers typically of the lower extremities. Osteomyelitis is a common complication of diabetic foot ulcers.

DIAGNOSTIC CRITERIA

Diagnosis of diabetes is based on: HbA1c $\geq$ 6.5%, or FBS > 125 mg/dl, or 2 hour OGTT > 200 mg/dl, or random glucose > 200 mg/dl + symptoms of hyperglycemia (e.g., polyuria, polydipsia, blurred vision).

Hyperglycemia: Blood sugar > 140 mg/dl

Hypoglycemia: Blood sugar < 70 mg/dl

Diabetic hyperglycemia hyperosmolar state (HHS): Characterized by severe hyperglycemia (blood sugar > 600), hyperosmolarity, dehydration without significant ketoacidosis, and usually some alteration in consciousness (coma if severe). Diagnostic criteria include:

- Blood sugar > 600 mg/dl
- Serum osmolality > 320 mmol/L
- Other findings: pH > 7.30, Bicarbonate > 18

Diabetic ketoacidosis (DKA): Characterized by hyperglycemia, acidosis, elevated serum ketones, and dehydration. Diagnostic criteria require all of the following:

- Blood sugar > 250 mg/dl
- Acidosis with pH < 7.30
- Bicarbonate < 18 mEq/L (HCO3 on BMP or ABG)
- Marked elevation of serum ketones (urinary ketones also elevated but not a diagnostic criterion)

Hyponatremia with diabetic hyperglycemia. In diabetic hyperglycemia, glucose dilutes sodium which makes the measured sodium level lower than it really is. Therefore, it's necessary to calculate a corrected sodium to get the true sodium value to determine if a patient has hyponatremia or hypernatremia (or a normal sodium level).

To calculate the corrected sodium level in patients with hyperglycemia, use measured sodium + 0.016 x (Glucose – 100) or an on-line calculator.

EXAMPLE 1 Glucose 700 with measured sodium 128 that falsely appears to be hyponatremia. The corrected sodium level = 137.6, which is normal and would be considered "pseudohyponatremia."
Calculation: 128 + 0.016 x 600 = 137.6.

EXAMPLE 2 Glucose 700 with measured sodium 142 (normal). The corrected sodium level is 151.6 (hypernatremia). Calculation: 142 + 0.016 x 600 = 151.6.

TREATMENT

Treatment of HHS and DKA is rather complicated and overlaps but includes insulin (usually starting with IV), IV fluids, correction of electrolyte imbalance, monitoring of response, and many other things depending on the clinical circumstances. Management of complications depends on the specific complication and its manifestations.

CODING AND DOCUMENTATION CHALLENGES

Although the chronic diabetic complications do not have CC status, all are included in CMS-HCC 18.

All of the diabetic complications listed in the ICD-10 Index and Tabular (except those indexed as "NEC") are automatically linked and the diabetes code can be assigned, unless specifically stated as unrelated (OCG I.A.15).

In most cases, a combination code identifies the type of diabetes and the complication. For "other specified" diabetic complications (E11.69), an additional code is also assigned for the complication.

According to Coding Clinic, the "**with**" guideline does not apply to diabetes codes with index entries that include "not elsewhere classified (NEC)" which cover broad categories of conditions, e.g., arthropathy NEC. If a **condition is not listed** as "with" diabetes or is listed as an "**NEC**" code in the index, the physician must establish a causal relationship.

To illustrate, a diabetic patient with a "skin ulcer" could not be coded as a diabetic skin ulcer. The skin ulcer would have to be linked to the diabetes by the provider. However, a foot ulcer is automatically linked to diabetes without provider clarification.

Terms that qualify for assignment to diabetes with **hyperglycemia** (E11.65) include out of control, inadequate control, or poorly controlled. "Uncontrolled" must be clarified as hyper- or hypoglycemia.

The term **type 1.5** has been used clinically to describe type 1 patients with insufficient insulin production who also have an element of peripheral insulin resistance characteristic of type 2. In this case, assign a code from category E13, other specified diabetes (Coding Clinic 2018 Third Quarter p.4).

Do not assign a code for hyponatremia in hyperglycemic patients with **pseudohyponatremia**. The low sodium would be considered an abnormal lab finding that is always inherent to the hyperglycemia. Be sure to calculate a corrected sodium (see above) to get the true sodium value to determine if a patient truly has hyponatremia or hypernatremia (or a normal sodium level).

Do not assign the ketoacidosis code for documentation of diabetic "**ketosis**." Even though this term is indexed to ketoacidosis, it is not a clinically valid diagnosis unless acidosis is present.

For **DRG Tips**, see DRG 637-638, Diabetes.

References

- Expert Committee on the Diagnosis and Classification of Diabetes Mellitus: Follow-up report on the diagnosis of diabetes mellitus. Diabetes Care: 2003; 26: 3160-3167
- WHO: Use of Glycated Haemoglobin (HbA1c) in the Diagnosis of Diabetes Mellitus
- UpToDate.com: Overview of medical care in adults with diabetes mellitus
- Medscape: Hyperosmolar Hyperglycemic State
- Diabetic Ketoacidosis: Evaluation and Treatment Am Fam Physician 2013;87: 337-346

- American Diabetes Association: Diabetic Ketoacidosis and Hyperglycemic Hyperosmolar Syndrome: Diabetes Spectrum 2002: 15: 28-36
- Coding Clinic 2018 Second Quarter p. 6
- Coding Clinic 2017 First Quarter p. 42
- Coding Clinic 2017 Fourth Quarter p. 100
- Coding Clinic 2016 Second Quarter p. 10, 30
- Coding Clinic 2020 First Quarter p. 15: Pseudohyponatremia.

DEFINITION

Electrolyte level above or below normal reference range that requires some form of management or intervention.

Includes sodium, potassium, calcium, magnesium, phosphate, bicarbonate and chloride. Abnormal bicarbonate and chloride are typically described as metabolic acidosis or alkalosis.

DIAGNOSTIC CRITERIA

Electrolytes above or below normal reference range (may vary slightly among labs). For example:

Sodium	134 – 146 meq/L
Metabolic alkalosis	Elevated bicarbonate >28 meq/L
Metabolic acidosis	Low bicarbonate <22 meq/L and/or elevated chloride > 106 meq/L

TREATMENT

The management of electrolyte abnormalities (hypo- and hyper-) involves correction to normal levels, at least daily monitoring, and in some cases EKG and cardiac monitoring for arrhythmias.

Low electrolyte levels (hypo-) are primarily treated with oral or IV replacement, correction of any underlying cause and discontinuation of contributory medications. For example, treatment of **hyponatremia** may involve oral sodium supplement, discontinue thiazide diuretics (e.g., HCTZ), fluid restriction or, if severe, 3% hypertonic saline (in contrast to normal saline which is 0.9%).

Management of high electrolyte levels (hyper-) is typically more complicated than low levels involving distinct types of treatment to reduce levels and manage or prevent complications. For example, treatment of **hypernatremia** may include discontinuing "loop" diuretics (e.g., Lasix, Bumex), IV D5W or 1/2 normal saline.

The treatment of **metabolic acidosis** and **alkalosis** depends entirely on its cause including correction or treatment of the underlying cause(s). For metabolic alkalosis, correction of hypovolemia and hypokalemia is commonly needed. In severe anion-gap acidosis, IV bicarbonate may be required.

SIADH is excessive secretion of anti-diuretic hormone (ADH) and characterized by hyponatremia that does not improve with treatment, low serum osmolality, and normal or elevated urine osmolality. Treatment consists of fluid restriction, discontinuing diuretics; hypertonic saline (3%) infusion may be necessary.

CODING AND DOCUMENTATION CHALLENGES

Codes for hyponatremia (E87.1), hypernatremia (E87.0), metabolic acidosis (E87.2), and metabolic alkalosis (E87.3) are CCs.

To permit code assignment, a provider must document the medical diagnostic term that describes the lab finding (do not code from the lab report). For example, low sodium = "hyponatremia."

Code assignment requires some form of intervention — treatment, monitoring, extended length of stay. Minimally increased or decreased electrolyte levels that require no attention would not be clinically significant.

In patients with **diabetic hyperglycemia**, a low sodium may be a pseudohyponatremia and a low or normal sodium may actually be hypernatremia — see "Hyponatremia with diabetic hyperglycemia" in *Diabetic Complications.*

For *DRG Tips,* see DRGs 640-641, Nutrition, metabolic, fluid/electrolyte disorders.

References

• UpToDate.com: Overview of the treatment of hyponatremia in adults; Treatment of hypernatremia; Treatment and prevention of hyperkalemia in adults.

DEFINITION

The National Institute of Neurologic Disorders and Stroke (NINDS) of the NIH describes encephalopathy as "any diffuse disease of the brain that alters brain function or structure." Encephalopathy can be further classified as acute (functional) or chronic (structural).

DIAGNOSTIC CRITERIA

Acute (functional) encephalopathy:
- Acute or subacute diffuse (generalized) alteration in brain function/mental status in the absence of a structural abnormality typically due to a systemic underlying cause
- Reversible and resolves when the underlying cause is corrected
- Structural changes do not occur

CT/MRI expected to be unremarkable since the brain abnormality is functional, not structural. EEG is usually unnecessary but may show diffuse slowing or low amplitude and can rule out subclinical seizures.

Chronic (structural) encephalopathy:
- Structural, irreversible due to permanent brain damage
- May be diffuse (generalized) or focal changes in brain function/ mental status

Chronic causes include traumatic, Korsakoff (alcohol), Binswanger (subcortical vascular dementia), spongiform (viral), chronic toxic (cumulative exposure to solvents or heavy metals), and various hereditary metabolic disorders.

Components of **mental status**: Alertness, attention, behavior, communication, judgement, memory, orientation, perception of reality, and thought content.

Specific Types of Acute Encephalopathy:

Metabolic (G93.41) due to such things as fever, dehydration, electrolyte imbalance, hypoglycemia, hypoxemia, infection, and organ failure.

Toxic (G92.9) refers to the effects of drugs and toxins.

Toxic-metabolic (G92.8) is a combination of toxic and metabolic factors.

Septic encephalopathy (G93.41) is a manifestation of severe sepsis, which is a specific type of metabolic encephalopathy.

Hepatic encephalopathy (K72.90) is due to elevated blood ammonia levels and describes a spectrum of neurologic impairment (e.g., altered mental status, combativeness) in patients with severe end-stage liver disease. See *Hepatic Encephalopathy & Failure.*

Hypertensive encephalopathy (I67.4) is an acute or subacute consequence of severe hypertension marked by headache, obtundation, confusion, or stupor, with or without convulsions. Papilledema may be noted.

Hypoxic ischemic encephalopathy, or **HIE** (P91.60) applies only to neonates and is an acute or subacute brain injury due to oxygen deprivation at delivery. Common in premature infants. Symptoms may include meconium-stained amniotic fluid, bradycardia, poor muscle tone, weak or no breathing, bluish or pale skin color, or acidosis. Seizures are a common manifestation. May cause permanent brain damage.

Neonatal encephalopathy (P91.819) is a syndrome of neurological dysfunction usually in full term newborns that involves depressed or disturbed neurological function often caused by lack of oxygen during birth.

Specific Types of Chronic Encephalopathy:

Alcoholic encephalopathy (G31.2) is permanent degeneration of the nervous system due to alcohol commonly involving the cerebellum.

Hypoxic or anoxic encephalopathy (G93.1) is permanent chronic brain damage due to sustained hypoxia.

Static encephalopathy (G93.49) is a term used to describe a patient with a chronic or permanent impairment of brain function, usually in children.

Wernicke's encephalopathy (E51.2) is manifested by acute oculomotor (eye muscle) dysfunction and ataxia caused by thiamine deficiency in alcoholics. Korsakoff syndrome is a late manifestation of Wernicke's associated with profound amnesia.

TREATMENT

Correction of underlying systemic cause(s), supportive care and safety measures, cautious use of antipsychotics like Haldol; lactulose for hepatic encephalopathy.

CODING AND DOCUMENTATION CHALLENGES

Encephalopathy is the underlying cause of an acute generalized alteration of mental status for most patients admitted to hospitals and commonly occurs in the elderly especially those with dementia. It is often the principal reason for admission (principal diagnosis) and a common comorbidity.

Encephalopathy is assigned as the principal diagnosis if it is the primary reason for inpatient admission. For example, patients with a UTI are often admitted mainly for encephalopathy (mental status alteration), not for the UTI itself. Uncomplicated UTIs can usually be treated as an outpatient or in observation; acute encephalopathy is a serious medical condition requiring inpatient care.

Because unspecified encephalopathy (G93.40) is a CC, it is essential that the specific type of encephalopathy be documented and if not, a query submitted to clarify.

Toxic encephalopathy refers to the effects of medications (drug-induced) and toxins. If due to a poisoning or toxin, the poisoning code (T36-T50) or toxic effect code (T51-T65) is sequenced first followed by the G92 code. If toxic encephalopathy is due to an adverse effect of medication, the G92 code is sequenced first followed by the adverse effect code (T36-T50).

An acute **toxic encephalopathy due to alcohol intoxication** is coded as T51.0X1A and G92.9 (MCC), not as alcoholic encephalopathy G31.2, a non-CC.

Intoxication delirium (F10.221) is likely to be consistent with a toxic encephalopathy due to alcohol but would require provider specification of the toxic encephalopathy. For example: "Intoxication delirium caused by toxic encephalopathy due to alcohol."

Withdrawal delirium (delirium tremens) is not a toxic encephalopathy since the toxin has actually been withdrawn. The correct code for this situation is F10.231 (alcohol dependence with withdrawal delirium).

Hypoxic or anoxic encephalopathy, code G93.1, represents permanent chronic brain damage and should not be assigned for a patient who has an acute functional metabolic encephalopathy temporarily due to hypoxemia which may need clarification by the provider.

Hepatic encephalopathy is coded to "hepatic failure" and is an MCC if documented as acute, subacute or with coma. Typically when a patient is admitted with hepatic encephalopathy, it is the principal diagnosis. See *Hepatic Encephalopathy & Failure*.

According to Coding Clinic 2021, a patient diagnosed with **toxic metabolic encephalopathy due to acute on chronic hepatic encephalopathy** would be assigned codes K7200 and K7210 for the acute and chronic hepatic encephalopathy (failure) and code G92.8 to specifically capture the toxic metabolic encephalopathy. Howevere, be aware that since metabolic encephalopathy is inherent to hepatic encephalopathy, this may not be clinically valid *unless* there is another condition causing the metabolic encephalopathy.

Encephalopathy due to diabetic hypoglycemia is assigned to code E11.649 and G93.41, an MCC, if specified as metabolic encephalopathy. If documented as unspecified "encephalopathy" (G93.40) or diabetic encephalopathy (G93.49), these are both classified as CCs.

Although "Encephalopathy, hypoglycemic" is indexed to code E16.2 (unspecified hypoglycemia), it is not with diabetes (see Excludes1 note).

Encephalopathy due to CVA. Coding Clinic 2017 Second Quarter, advised to "Assign code G93.49, other encephalopathy, for encephalopathy that occurs secondary to an acute cerebrovascular accident/stroke. Although the encephalopathy is associated with an acute lacunar infarct, it is not inherent, and therefore is coded when it occurs."

Coding Clinic did not address whether such a diagnosis would be a clinically valid one since Coding Clinic disclaims any authority for clinical diagnostic definitions or standards. Since encephalopathy represents a generalized alteration of mental status in the absence of structural abnormality, the clinical validity of "encephalopathy due to CVA" could be challenged.

Delirium vs. encephalopathy. The terms delirium and encephalopathy describe essentially the same set of clinical circumstances. However, ICD-10 classifies delirium (CC or non-CC) as a mental disorder or a symptom; encephalopathy (often an MCC) is recognized as a specific medical condition that may cause delirium.

The Diagnostic and Statistical Manual of Mental Disorders, Fifth Edition (DSM-5), developed and published by the American Psychiatric Association, is the authoritative source for classification of mental disorders. It does not address the diagnostic term "encephalopathy" because this is considered a medical condition, not a mental disorder.

DSM-5 defines delirium as "a disturbance in attention and awareness that develops over a short time…not occur[ring] in the context of severely reduced level of arousal, such as coma." It further classifies delirium as due to drug/chemical intoxication or withdrawal or as "attributable to the physiological consequences of another medical condition."

DSM-5 states "The other medical condition should also be coded and listed separately immediately before delirium…(e.g., K72.90 hepatic encephalopathy)." This is a clear instruction by DSM-5 to also document the underlying cause of delirium (such as toxic or metabolic encephalopathy) and code it first. Examples are "Toxic encephalopathy due to Dilantin causing delirium" or "Delirium due to metabolic encephalopathy."

This approach by DSM-5 is consistent with ICD-10 as well as the fact that encephalopathy encompasses delirium and other states of altered mental status. ICD-10 Tabular instructions for code F05, Delirium due to known physiological condition: "Code first the underlying physiological condition"—as for example encephalopathy.

If only delirium is documented, a query for encephalopathy as the cause would generally be warranted if substantiated by clinical criteria.

Dementia and encephalopathy. A commonly encountered dilemma is establishing and validating the diagnosis of encephalopathy when a patient with preexisting dementia is admitted with an altered mental status. Sudden changes in mental functioning are not expected with most progressive dementias and require prompt medical attention.

This distinction should be relatively simple. A patient with dementia has encephalopathy when a genuine acute or subacute mental status alteration associated with metabolic or toxic factors occurs and improves or returns to baseline status when the causative factors are corrected. Nursing notes may help clarify whether a genuine change occurred.

If no toxic or metabolic factors are evident, or if the patient's mental status does not improve during hospitalization, encephalopathy is unlikely.

Patients with dementia may experience **sundowning** which describes a patient with agitation, anxiety, or confusion that occurs during the late afternoon or evening. Code F05, Delirium due to known physiological condition, a CC, is assigned for sundowning.

Although **encephalopathy with influenza** is indexed to code J11.81, this code would only be assigned when the influenza is due to an unidentified influenza virus.

For *DRG Tips*, see DRGs 70-72, Non-specific cerebrovascular disorders.

References

- UpToDate.com: Acute toxic-metabolic encephalopathy in adults
- UpToDate.com: Diagnosis of delirium and confusional states
- UpToDate.com: Hepatic encephalopathy in adults: Clinical manifestations and diagnosis
- National Institute of Neurologic Disorders and Stroke: NINDS Encephalopathy Information
- Coding Clinic 2016 Second Quarter p. 35
- Coding Clinic 2017 Second Quarter p. 9
- Coding Clinic 2021 First Quarter p. 13

DEFINITION

Excisional debridement is the surgical removal or cutting away of devitalized tissue, necrosis, or slough using a scalpel or curette, not scissors.

Non-excisional debridement is the cleaning, brushing, scrubbing, washing, irrigating of a wound; chemical or enzymatic treatment; or minor trimming/scraping to remove fragments of dead tissue.

Excisional biopsy is the surgical removal of a whole lesion or mass. This is in contrast to an incisional biopsy which is when only a tissue sample is excised from a mass and removed for diagnosis.

CODING AND DOCUMENTATION CHALLENGES

In every case of wound or decubitus care, review for documentation of debridement in the progress notes or operative report.

Debridement can be performed or documented by any provider who is licensed and credentialed to perform this procedure, including healthcare professionals like nurses, physician assistants, podiatrists. It can be performed in the OR, ED, minor procedure area, or bedside.

Excisional debridement is classified as the root operation "Excision" and is considered an OR procedure that impacts DRG assignment even if performed at the bedside.

For clarity, the term **excisional**, excised, or excision should be documented; and/or the documentation meets the root operation definition of "cutting out or off, without replacement, a portion of a body part" per Coding Clinic. Scissors should not be used for excisional debridement because they cause tissue trauma by crushing healthy tissue.

"**Sharply debrided**" indicates than an excision was performed but must be clarified as excisional.

EXCISIONAL DEBRIDEMENT / BIOPSY

Non-excisional debridement is classified as the root operation "extraction" and has no impact on DRG assignment. The use of Versa-Jet without additional surgical "cutting away" of tissue is classified by ICD-10-PCS as non-excisional debridement.

Physicians are sometimes perplexed because CPT-4 procedural coding does not require documentation of "excisional," and the hospital's need to correctly classify the procedure using ICD-10-PCS should be explained.

An "**excisional biopsy**" of an entire mass or lesion is also classified as an "excision" when it is completely excised. It should be coded with a 7th digit of Z and not coded with 7th digit X "diagnostic" for biopsy. For example, "excisional biopsy" of left thigh abscess that was completely excised is coded as 0JBM0ZZ and considered an OR procedure.

Sometimes during an incision and drainage (I&D), the provider may also perform excisional debridement of "**necrotic**" tissue. Necrotic/necrosis is coded to gangrene (I96) if not elsewhere classified; if with diabetes is coded to E11.52, which are CCs. Review the operative report carefully and query if clarification is necessary.

Remember also that any debridement procedure is classified based on its greatest **depth** and that different levels of debridement are assigned to different ICD-10-PCS code categories (some impacting the DRG and some not): skin, subcutaneous tissue/fascia, muscle, bone, joint, tendon, ligament/bursa. Most excisional debridements are of the subcutaneous tissue or deeper. If coded to excision of "skin" it will not be classified as an OR procedure.

For **DRG Tips,** see DRGs 570-572, Skin debridement.

References

- Coding Clinic 2014 Third Quarter p. 14
- Coding Clinic 2015 First Quarter p. 23
- Coding Clinic 2015 Third Quarter p. 3
- Coding Clinic 2018 Third Quarter p. 3.

135

DEFINITION

Functional quadriplegia (R53.2) is the inability to use one's limbs and ambulate due to extreme debility caused by another medical condition without physical injury or damage to the spinal cord.

The terms quadriplegia or quadriparesis (less than total paralysis) are typically used for the consequences of upper spinal cord injury.

DIAGNOSTIC CRITERIA

Typically the patient requires "total care." The usual findings are: bedridden, inability to turn, unable to feed or groom self, urinary/fecal incontinence, flexion contractures.

Braden scores:
- Mobility = 1 (completely immobile) or 2 (very limited)
- Activity = 1 (bedridden)

ADLs: High degree of disability or dependence, incontinence, complete immobility. Not simply "needs assistance."

Common causes:

- Severe, end-stage dementia
- Advanced progressive neuro-degenerative disorders (e.g., multiple sclerosis, ALS, cerebral palsy, Huntington's disease)
- Severe brain injury/brain damage
- Advanced musculoskeletal deformity, severe crippling arthritis
- Profound intellectual disability

Functional quadriplegia is an MCC and highly-weighted CMS-HCC, as is structural (spinal) quadriplegia.

References
- CMS Open Door Forum (2/14/13): Clarification related to active diagnoses and quadriplegia.

DEFINITION

Heart failure is defined as inadequate cardiac output resulting from functional or structural abnormalities of the heart. It is a clinical diagnosis based on the Framingham Clinical Criteria which uses a number of major and minor criteria. Causes include coronary artery disease (CAD), hypertension, valvular heart disease, myocarditis, congenital heart defects, among others.

Common symptoms include shortness of breath (dyspnea) at rest or with exertion, orthopnea, nocturnal dyspnea or cough, and easy fatigability.

DIAGNOSTIC CRITERIA

Systolic Heart Failure (HFrEF)
- Heart failure with left ventricular ejection fraction (LVEF) < 50%
- Most common cause is ischemic heart disease, e.g., CAD

Diastolic Heart Failure (HFpEF)
- Heart failure with left ventricular ejection fraction ≥ 50%
- Echo may also show "diastolic dysfunction" parameters
- Most common cause is hypertension and/or ESRD

Combined Systolic/Diastolic
- Heart failure with ejection fraction < 50% + evidence of diastolic dysfunction on echo

Indicators of acute heart failure:
- Exacerbation of symptoms
- Physical exam: rales and/or increasing edema
- IV medications (usually Lasix)
- Pulmonary edema/congestion or increasing (or new) pleural effusion on chest x-ray
- BNP > 500 or NT-proBNP based on age (if no renal impairment): > 450 (Age < 50), > 900 (Age 50-75), > 1,800 (Age > 75)
- Hypoxemia / need for supplemental oxygen

TREATMENT

Diuretics: Lasix (furosemide), Bumex (bumetanide),* Zaroxolyn (metolazone),* Aldactone (spironolactone)

Beta-blockers: Coreg (carvedilol)–almost exclusively for heart failure, Lopressor/Toprol (metoprolol),* Zebeta (bisoprolol)*

ACE inhibitors (ACEI)*: Prinivil/Zestril (lisinopril), Vasotec (enalapril), Capoten (captopril)

Angiotensin receptor blockers (ARB)*: Cozaar (losartan), Avapro (irbesartan), Diovan (valsartan), Micardis (telmisartan)

Digoxin
- Used for systolic heart failure only (not diastolic)
- Also used to control ventricular rate in atrial fibrillation when LVEF <40%

Nitrates for severe systolic heart failure (usually not diastolic)
- Nitroglycerin (IV, transdermal, oral)
- Imdur (isosorbide mononitrite)
- Isordil (isosorbide dinitrate)

Hydralazine*: arterial vasodilator frequently combined with nitrates for severe systolic heart failure

These drugs are also used for hypertension.

CODING AND DOCUMENTATION CHALLENGES

When heart failure is principal diagnosis, the specification of systolic or diastolic failure does not change the DRG or severity classification. As a secondary diagnosis, heart failure must be specified as:

1. Systolic or diastolic (CC), and
2. Acute (MCC) or chronic/unspecified (CC)

Stable, chronic, asymptomatic heart failure is a CC, but only if specified as systolic or diastolic.

The physician should not be queried for acuity unless the patient meets the indicators for acute heart failure (see above). Terms like **decompensated** and **exacerbation** are equivalent to acute.

Physicians may be more inclined clinically to recognize and acknowledge a decompensation or exacerbation (especially when mild) than to document "acute" which may imply an acute, severe situation to them. Including these terms in a multiple-choice query option allows the provider to more accurately portray the true severity of illness in such cases. Giving one or more doses of IV Lasix promptly would be expected to justify or validate the diagnosis.

Heart failure with **reduced** ejection fraction, HFrEF, is defined as heart failure with an ejection fraction < 40% and indexed to systolic heart failure. Heart failure with preserved ejection fraction, HFpEF, is defined as heart failure with an ejection fraction ≥ 50% and indexed to diastolic heart failure.

Recently the term heart failure with "**mid-range**" or "**mildly reduced**" ejection fraction (HFmrEF) defined as EF 41–49% has been introduced.

Heart failure with **recovered** ejection fraction (HFrecEF) or **improved** ejection fraction (HFimpEF) is significant improvement of reduced EF (systolic heart failure) usually following aortic valve replacement such as TAVR. Significant improvement is defined as a baseline EF < 40% with a 10% or more increase resulting in a new baseline > 40%. For example, baseline of 35% that increased 12% to 47%.

Coding Clinic 2020 Third Quarter, p. 32, advises to code chronic systolic heart failure for patients with heart failure described with reduced, mildly reduced, or mid-range ejection fraction, and to code chronic diastolic heart failure for patients with a recovered EF that is normal (≥ 50%). If the EF does not recover to normal, a query may be necessary to determine if the recovered EF represents systolic or diastolic failure.

Other terms for systolic heart failure may include heart failure "with low EF" or "with reduced systolic function." Diastolic heart failure may include heart failure "with preserved ventricular function" or "preserved systolic function." Whenever these or similar terms are used, the coder may interpret these as systolic heart failure or diastolic heart failure.

The term "hypertensive cardiomyopathy with preserved ventricular function" may be used to describe diastolic heart failure, but because heart failure isn't mentioned it needs to be clarified whether it is diastolic heart failure or not.

Coding Clinic First Quarter 2017 indicates that **systolic or diastolic dysfunction must be linked to heart failure** by the provider to be assigned as systolic or diastolic heart failure. Otherwise, assign code I50.9 (unspecified heart failure).

Subcategory I50.8-- includes various types of acute and chronic right heart failure, biventricular, high-output and end-stage heart failure all of which are non-CCs. The codes have no systolic or diastolic specificity so it's necessary to get that specificity to allow assignment of those codes that are CC/MCCs. Remember that all forms of heart failure documented are to be coded.

Example: Acute diastolic right heart failure. Assign codes I50.31 (acute diastolic heart failure) and I50.811 (acute right heart failure).

When **pleural effusion** is associated with heart failure, it is not separately coded unless it requires specific evaluation (such as chest x-rays or CT scan), treatment (like therapeutic thoracentesis) or is attributed to another condition by the provider.

ESRD and heart failure. When ESRD patients are admitted with CHF due to fluid overload and noncompliance with dialysis treatment, CHF is assigned as the principal diagnosis.

Fluid overload should be assigned as principal diagnosis when a patient is admitted with fluid overload due to dialysis non-compliance and the patient has (1) no history or evidence of CHF, or (2) a history of CHF but the provider specifically indicates the fluid overload was non-cardiogenic in nature and the CHF was not decompensated.

Hypertensive heart and kidney disease. In patients admitted principally for acute heart failure but who also have hypertension and CKD (cardio-renal syndrome) the hypertensive heart and CKD code (I13.0) is assigned as principal diagnosis and the acute heart failure (MCC) becomes a secondary diagnosis. According to OCG I.C.9.a, the causal relationship between the three conditions is assumed, unless the documentation clearly states the conditions are unrelated.

For **DRG Tips**, see DRGs 291-293, Heart failure & shock.

References

• Universal Definition and Classification of Heart Failure. J Card Fail 2021;27:387-413.

• 2013 ACCF/AHA Guideline for the Management of Heart Failure. Executive summary: A Report of the American College of Cardiology Foundation/American Heart Association Task Force on Practice Guidelines. J Am Coll Cardiol 2013; 62:1495–1539

• McKee, PA et al. The Natural History of Congestive Heart Failure: The Framingham Study. N Engl J Med 1971; 85:1441-1446

• Heart Failure with Mid-Range Ejection Fraction – a New Category of Heart Failure or Still a Gray Zone. Maedica (Buchar). 2016; 11: 320–324

• Early Recovery of Left Ventricular Systolic Function After CoreValve Transcatheter Aortic Valve Replacement. Circ Cardiovasc Interv. 2016; 9: e003425

• Januzzi, JL et al. NT-proBNP testing for diagnosis and short-term prognosis in acute destabilized heart failure: an international pooled analysis of 1256 patients. Eur Heart J 2006; 27: 330-37

• www.emedicine.medscape: Heart Failure Treatment & Management

• UpToDate.com: Natriuretic peptide measurement in heart failure

• Coding Clinic 2007 Third Quarter p. 11

• Coding Clinic 2016 First Quarter p. 10

• Coding Clinic 2017 First Quarter p. 46

• Coding Clinic 2020 Third Quarter p. 32.

DEFINITION

The liver is the largest solid organ in the body and part of the digestive system. It carries out hundreds of essential tasks including detoxification (bilirubin, alcohol, medications), protein synthesis (albumin), blood clotting (prothrombin), and the production of bile that breaks down fats during digestion.

Hepatic (liver) failure is a life-threatening condition that occurs when the liver is damaged and no longer able to function properly. Liver failure can happen suddenly (acute) or develop slowly over time (chronic), depending on the cause.

Acute hepatic failure refers to the development of severe acute liver injury (identified by liver test abnormalities) with encephalopathy and prolonged prothrombin time (INR of ≥1.5) in patients without cirrhosis or pre-existing liver disease. Common causes of acute liver failure are acetaminophen toxicity, drugs and toxins (e.g., mushroom poisoning), viral hepatitis, malignancy, sepsis, severe hypotension ("shock liver").

Chronic hepatic failure is most common and usually due to cirrhosis which is marked by destruction of liver cells, chronic inflammation, and fibrosis. Cirrhosis is typically a result of alcohol abuse, hepatitis B or C, or non-alcoholic fatty liver disease (NAFLD). Complications of cirrhosis include ascites, hepatic encephalopathy, spontaneous bacterial peritonitis, secondary renal failure (hepatorenal syndrome), and portal hypertension.

Hepatic encephalopathy describes a spectrum of neurologic impairment in patients with liver failure such as altered mental status, confusion, disorientation, inappropriate behavior, combativeness, gait disturbances, and/or altered level of consciousness ranging from drowsiness to deep coma. An elevated level of neurotoxic blood ammonia confirms the diagnosis, and it is treated with lactulose. Hepatic encephalopathy can be acute (overt), chronic, or acute on chronic.

Liver failure is classified based on how long the patient has been ill: hyperacute (< 7 days), acute (7 to 21 days), subacute (> 21 days and < 26 weeks), and chronic (> 26 weeks).

Chronic Liver Failure	Acute Liver Failure
Patients usually have cirrhosis resulting from alcohol abuse, hepatitis B or C, or non-alcoholic fatty liver disease.	Patients typically do not have cirrhosis or pre-existing liver disease. Common causes are acetaminophen toxicity, drugs and toxins, viral hepatitis, malignancy, sepsis, severe hypotension ("shock liver").
Diagnostic Criteria: Abnormal laboratory tests: • Elevated aminotransferase (AST & ALT), • Elevated bilirubin, or • Low platelet count (< 150K) Ascites, hepatorenal syndrome, and portal hypertension are often associated.	Diagnostic Criteria: Prolonged and progressively increasing prothrombin time: INR of ≥ 1.5. Other abnormal laboratory tests: • Elevated aminotransferase (AST & ALT), • Elevated bilirubin, or • Low platelet count (< 150K)

DIAGNOSTIC CRITERIA

The definitive diagnostic criteria for acute hepatic failure is a prolonged and progressively increasing prothrombin time:

- INR of ≥1.5 (in the absence of Vitamin K treatment).

Abnormal laboratory tests typically found in liver failure include:

- Elevated aminotransferase (AST & ALT)
- Elevated bilirubin
- Low platelet count (< 150K)

Other laboratory and clinical findings for liver failure include elevated creatinine, amylase/lipase, GGT, alkaline phosphatase, LDH; low pre-albumin/albumin; anemia.

Physical findings include jaundice, hepatomegaly, RUQ/liver tenderness, ascites/edema, and asterixis (rhythmic "flapping" of hands when wrists held fully extended).

TREATMENT

Treatment includes management of underlying cause and any complications, lactulose for hepatic encephalopathy, vitamin K, avoidance of hepatotoxic drugs, N-acetylcysteine for acetaminophen toxicity, and liver transplant for the most severe cases.

CODING AND DOCUMENTATION CHALLENGES

Although hepatic encephalopathy and hepatic failure are different clinical entities, they are both assigned to code K72.90, Hepatic failure, a non-CC. Acute hepatic encephalopathy and acute hepatic failure are assigned to K72.00, Acute and subacute hepatic failure—unless the acute hepatic failure is due to alcohol (K70.40), toxic liver disease (K71.10), or is postprocedural (K91.82). Chronic hepatic encephalopathy and chronic hepatic failure are both assigned to code K72.10, Chronic hepatic failure.

When a patient is admitted with hepatic encephalopathy due to chronic liver cirrhosis (underlying condition), hepatic encephalopathy (the acute manifestation) would be assigned as the principal diagnosis. Cirrhosis is usually not assigned as the principal diagnosis except in patients admitted for surgical intervention since it is a chronic condition. For patients admitted with bleeding esophageal varices due to cirrhosis, the cirrhosis is principal diagnosis based on the etiology/manifestation coding guideline. See *Cause and Effect.*

Hepatic encephalopathy and hepatic failure are non-CCs. Hepatic failure specified as "acute", "subacute", or "with coma" are MCCs if a secondary diagnosis. Hepatic encephalopathy and hepatic failure should be clinically validated based on the diagnostic criteria included above.

Review for indicators of "**coma**", such as GCS total score of 8 or less, abnormal EEG, and documentation of unconsciousness, stupor, obtundation. See *Coma.*

"Shock liver", also known as ischemic hepatitis, is a term that describes acute liver failure due to severe hypotension, i.e., shock.

According to Coding Clinic 2021 First Quarter, p. 13, a patient diagnosed with **toxic metabolic encephalopathy due to acute on chronic hepatic encephalopathy** would be assigned codes K72.00 and K72.10 for the acute and chronic hepatic encephalopathy (failure) and code G92.8 to specifically capture the toxic metabolic encephalopathy. Although there are no excludes notes that prohibit coding G92.8 or G93.41 with hepatic encephalopathy, metabolic encephalopathy is inherent to hepatic encephalopathy so it may not be clinically valid unless there is another condition causing the metabolic encephalopathy.

A diagnosis of "**acute liver injury**" should not be assigned to injury code S36.119A if there was no traumatic injury to the liver. Per Coding Clinic, a diagnosis of "acute liver injury" with "acute hepatitis" should be assigned to code K72.00 (acute and subacute hepatitis failure without coma). If the cause of the liver injury is unknown, the provider should be queried.

In cases where the underlying cause is not included as part of the hepatic failure code, the underlying cause should also be coded. For example, chronic viral hepatitis C (B18.2) with chronic hepatic failure (K72.10). Sequencing depends on the circumstances of the admission.

Liver failure as principal diagnosis is assigned to two DRG triplets: 432-434 (Cirrhosis & alcoholic hepatitis) and 441-443 (Disorders of the liver except malignancy, cirrhosis, alcoholic hepatitis). The DRG relative weights are not substantially different.

References

- UpToDate.com: Acute liver failure in adults: Etiology, clinical manifestations, and diagnosis
- UpToDate.com: Acute liver failure in adults: Management and prognosis
- UpToDate.com: Cirrhosis in adults: Etiologies, clinical manifestations, and diagnosis
- MELD Score Calculator: Stratifies severity of end-stage liver disease
- Coding Clinic 2002 First Quarter p. 3
- Coding Clinic 2015 Second Quarter p. 17.

DEFINITION

HIV disease, or AIDS, is caused by HIV (human immunodeficiency virus), all types, with destruction of CD4+ T-lymphocytes that help mediate the body's immune response to infection.

DIAGNOSTIC CRITERIA

The CDC is responsible for establishing the definitive case definitions of HIV infection and HIV disease (AIDS).

HIV infection (HIV-positive without AIDS) is defined by two different HIV antibody or antigen/antibody tests, or by non-antibody virologic testing (e.g., HIV culture).

HIV disease / AIDS for adults, adolescents and children > 18 months of age is defined as an HIV-positive patient who has or has had either of the following:

- Absolute CD4+ T-lymphocyte count < 200, or
- An AIDS-defining condition

AIDS-defining conditions: Common ones include pneumocystis pneumonia, certain lymphomas, systemic candidiasis, other unusual bacterial, fungal, parasitic, viral infections, and HIV wasting syndrome. A few AIDS-defining conditions apply only to children <13 years or only to adults and adolescents. The full list is available on the CDC website.

TREATMENT

The CDC recommends treatment with highly active antiretroviral therapy (HAART) of all HIV-positive patients, with or without AIDS. Therefore, treatment does not distinguish HIV-positive from AIDS.

CODING AND DOCUMENTATION CHALLENGES

The CDC recommends the use of the term **HIV disease** to describe AIDS. HIV illness is sometimes used and coded as AIDS.

The term "HIV infection" describes an HIV positive person who does not yet meet the diagnostic criteria for HIV disease.

Physicians often only document the ambiguous terms "HIV" or "HIV positive." ICD-10 classifies these terms as asymptomatic HIV (code Z21). Therefore, the provider's diagnostic intent must be clarified and clinically valid.

For every encounter, the clinically correct distinction between HIV disease vs. HIV-positive must be made. It also has profound implications for the HIV-positive patient who may or may not have progressed to HIV disease.

HIV disease / AIDS (code B20). If AIDS or HIV disease has ever been previously diagnosed and code B20 assigned, it must always be coded B20 on every subsequent encounter and never again code Z21. According to OCG Section I.C.1.a.2.f: "Patients with any known *prior* diagnosis of an HIV-related [AIDS-defining] illness should be coded to B20." If a patient with a history of HIV disease is currently managed on **antiretroviral** medications, assign code B20.

If the provider has only documented HIV, HIV+, or HIV infection and any prior records or other information indicates a diagnosis of AIDS or previous assignment of code B20, it must be brought to the attention of the provider for confirmation and correct coding of B20.

Proper terms for code B20 include HIV disease (preferred term), HIV illness, AIDS, ARC (AIDS-related complex), and HIV infection symptomatic. "Symptomatic" means any current or prior AIDS-defining condition.

HIV positive (code Z21). Used when the patient has never been diagnosed with AIDS or an AIDS-defining condition. Documentation that is coded Z21: HIV, HIV+, HIV infection, and HIV asymptomatic status (no current or prior AIDS-defining condition).

Only confirmed cases of HIV are coded, not probable or suspected.

When a patient is admitted with a diagnosis of HIV disease/AIDS (B20) and a major related condition (e.g., pneumonia) or other related condition, it will be grouped to an HIV DRG 969-977 regardless of whether B20 is a principal or a secondary diagnosis.

When a patient with AIDS is admitted for a condition that is not listed as one of the major related or other related conditions, the principal diagnosis is the **unrelated condition** and is assigned to the DRG for that condition, and B20 is coded as a secondary diagnosis (a CC).

Major related conditions include pneumonia, encephalopathy, sepsis, endocarditis, lymphomas, histoplasmosis, candidasis, cryptococcus, cytomegalovirus (CMV), toxoplasmosis, myelitis, herpes (zoster and some simplex), organic mental disorders, salmonella, TB (any type).

Other related conditions include lymphadenopathy, volume depletion, dehydration, fatigue/malaise, splenomegaly, thrombocytopenia, malnutrition, cachexia, gastroenteritis/colitis, dyspnea, febrile conditions (some), nephrotic syndrome.

EXAMPLES
- AIDS patient admitted for pneumonia. The DRG assigned is 976 AIDS with Major Related Condition [pneumonia] without CC/MCC. AIDS drives the DRG whether listed as principal or secondary diagnosis, and pneumonia is excluded as an MCC in this situation.

- AIDS patient admitted for dehydration. The DRG assigned is 977 AIDS with or w/o other related condition [dehydration].

- AIDS patient admitted for hip fracture requiring total hip replacement. The principal diagnosis is hip fracture with AIDS as CC and assigned to DRG 470 Major joint replacement of lower extremity w/o MCC.

References
- CDC: Revised Surveillance Case Definition for HIV Infection—United States, 2014, including Appendix A: AIDS-Defining Conditions
- Official Coding Guidelines I.C.1.a
- Coding Clinic 2019 First Quarter p. 8.

DEFINITION

Hypertensive crisis is a non-specific, general term for severe elevation of blood pressure (usually systolic BP >180 mmHg or diastolic BP >120 mmHg) intended to encompass both hypertensive urgency and emergency.

Hypertensive urgency is a severe elevation of blood pressure in otherwise stable patients requiring prompt intervention to gradually lower blood pressure.

Hypertensive emergency is severe elevation of blood pressure representing a more serious, potentially life-threatening condition requiring aggressive intervention to immediately lower blood pressure.

DIAGNOSTIC CRITERIA

Hypertensive urgency: severe blood pressure elevation usually in otherwise stable patients who may have symptoms such as headache, dyspnea, or non-specific chest pain without end-organ involvement.

Hypertensive emergency: severe blood pressure elevation with end-organ involvement.

End-organ involvement may include:
- Cardiovascular—heart failure, unstable angina, myocardial infarction
- Neurologic—hypertensive encephalopathy, seizure, stroke, brain hemorrhage
- Renal—acute kidney injury
- Eclampsia

TREATMENT

Hypertensive urgency: Gradual reduction of blood pressure over hours or days using typical oral antihypertensives (e.g., Atenolol, Lopressor, Lisinopril, Avapro, and many others). Aggressive immediate reduction is not recommended.

Hypertensive emergency: Immediate, urgent reduction using IV anti-hypertensives (e.g. , nitroprusside, nitroglycerin, labetalol, nicardipine, esmolol, hydralazine).

CODING AND DOCUMENTATION CHALLENGES

ICD-10 includes codes using current, accepted terminology:

- Hypertensive urgency (I16.0)—a non-CC
- Hypertensive emergency (I16.1)—a CC
- Hypertensive crisis (I16.9)—a CC

Outdated terms such as malignant and accelerated are non-essential modifiers resulting in code I10 (essential hypertension), a non-CC.

It is now particularly important to clarify whether a diagnosis of hypertensive urgency (non-CC) actually meets criteria for the more serious circumstances of hypertensive emergency (CC). Hypertensive crisis (CC) may be used to describe either emergency (CC) or urgency (non-CC).

Physicians may have to "unlearn" the old terminology of accelerated and malignant hypertension. If these terms are used, a query to clarify whether their use of accelerated or malignant hypertension actually represents either type of hypertensive crisis.

References

- JNC-7 (The Seventh Report of the Joint National Committee on Prevention, Detection, Evaluation, and Treatment of High Blood Pressure). JAMA 2003; 289 (19): 2560–2572
- 2017 ACC/AHA/AAPA/ABC/ACPM/AGS/APhA/ASH/ASPC/NMA/PCNA Guideline for the Prevention, Detection, Evaluation, and Management of High Blood Pressure in Adults. Hypertension 2018; 71:1269-1324.

Injuries and traumatic fractures are included in ICD-10-CM Chapter 19 Injury, Poisoning, and Certain Other Consequences of External Causes (S00–T88).

Traumatic injury codes should not be assigned for iatrogenic injuries that occur during or as a result of a **medical intervention**. Assign the appropriate complication code(s) instead.

Fractures can be open (open wound or break in skin near the site of the broken bone) or closed (skin is intact). Fracture codes specify the specific anatomical site, fracture type (e.g., greenstick, transverse, oblique, spiral, comminuted, segmental), displaced/nondisplaced, laterality, routine versus delayed healing, nonunion, and malunion.

Most codes that describe injuries require a 7th character to designate the encounter as initial, subsequent, or sequela which is important for accurate DRG assignment:

Initial encounter (A,B): Used while the patient is undergoing active treatment during an episode of care for the injury. Multiple physicians may assign the initial encounter when the visit is for active treatment of the initial injury. This might extend over several encounters.

Subsequent encounter (D,G,K,P): Used after the patient has received active treatment of the injury and is receiving routine care for the injury during the healing and recovery phase, i.e., cast change or removal, removal of internal/external fixation device, x-ray to check healing status of fracture, medication adjustment, other aftercare.

Sequela (S): Used for complications or conditions that arise as a direct result of an injury. The S extension identifies the injury responsible for the sequela. The specific type of sequela (e.g., scar, pain) is sequenced first, followed by the injury code with S as the 7th character. Sequela is the new term for late effects.

Initial vs. subsequent should be easily recognized from the medical record documentation and assigned on that basis if not specifically documented. A query might prompt an incorrect response since physicians are unlikely to understand the coding definitions of initial vs. subsequent.

Defaults (if not specified / documented):

- Displaced vs. non-displaced: Displaced
- Closed vs. open: Closed
- Healing: Routine
- Sequela: None
- Laterality: Unspecified side

Although laterality defaults to unspecified side, it should not be needed since laterality is always indicated somewhere in the inpatient medical record.

Gustilo type. Open fractures of the forearm, femur, lower leg, and ankle are further specified by the Gustilo fracture classification. A distinction only needs to be made between low-grade fractures (Gustilo I or II) and high-grade fractures (III):

- I or II: Small or low-energy wounds without major soft tissue damage or defect.
  Example: open fracture of tibia with clean 2 cm laceration.

- III (A,B,C): High-energy wounds with extensive soft tissue damage including muscle, skin, and neurovascular structures.
  Example: open fracture of femur with 12 cm wound and dermal loss with laceration of quadriceps muscle.

According to OCG section I.C.19.c.1, when the Gustilo type is not specified for an open fracture, type I or II should be assigned. Always query the provider if the documentation appears to support a Gustilo III fracture type.

References
- Official Coding Guidelines Sections I.C.19.a and I.C.19.c
- Coding Clinic 2015 First Quarter p. 3
- Coding Clinic 2016 First Quarter p. 33.

DEFINITION

Intellectual disability, formerly known as mental retardation, is characterized by:

- Impairment of intellectual function (IQ < 70)
- Associated with adaptive behavior problems
- Beginning prior to age 18

Adaptive behavior includes conceptual skills such as language, literacy, self-direction; social skills; and practical skills like activities of daily living, occupation and safety.

Borderline intellectual functioning (IQ 70–84) is considered a learning disability.

Classification of Intellectual Disability Severity

Severity	IQ Range (DSM-4 criteria)	DSM-5 Criteria	ICD-10 Code
Mild	Approximate IQ range 50-69	Can live independently with minimum levels of support	F70
Moderate	Approximate IQ range 36-49	Independent living with moderate levels of support, such as group homes	F71
Severe	Approximate IQ range 20-35	Requires daily assistance with self-care activities and safety supervision.	F72 (CC)
Profound	IQ < 20	Requires 24-hour care	F73 (CC)

Common Causes. Down's syndrome, cerebral palsy, autism, birth defects, fetal alcohol syndrome, infection, head trauma, and drugs, poisons, toxins.

Many patients with autism and cerebral palsy do not have intellectual disability.

CODING AND DOCUMENTATION CHALLENGES

Mental retardation is indexed as intellectual disability. Severity and/or the associated IQ should be documented for SOI and CC status. The underlying cause of intellectual disability should also be identified and coded as a separate diagnosis.

Potential comorbidity:

- Functional quadriplegia
- Pressure ulcers
- Encephalopathy—metabolic or toxic
- Aspiration pneumonia

References

- CDC: Developmental disabilities, specific conditions and Intellectual Disability Fact Sheet (www.cdc.gov/ncbddd
- US Dept of Education Center for Parent Information and Resources: Disabilities (www.parentcenterhub.org)
- American Association of Intellectual and Developmental Disabilities: Definition of Intellectual Disability and FAQ on Intellectual Disabilities (www.aaidd.org)
- The Arc: Intellectual Disability (www.thearc.org).

DEFINITION

The World Health Organization (WHO) refers to malnutrition as deficiencies, excesses or imbalances in a person's intake of energy and/or nutrients. The term malnutrition covers two broad groups of conditions: (1) "undernutrition" which includes stunting (low height for age), wasting (low weight for height), underweight (low weight for age) and micronutrient deficiencies or insufficiencies (a lack of important vitamins and minerals); and (2) overweight, obesity, and diet-related noncommunicable diseases (such as heart disease, stroke, diabetes and cancer).

DIAGNOSTIC CRITERIA

Prior to 2012, the diagnosis of malnutrition depended on a physician's subjective clinical judgment taking into account the number and severity of certain physical and clinical findings, such as: chronic disease (cancer, end-stage disease, alcoholism), physical findings (cachexia, muscle/adipose wasting), body mass composition (low body weight, unintended weight loss), and serum markers (low albumin, prealbumin, transferrin, cholesterol).

The limitations of this approach are subjectivity, lack of validating research, and multiple definitions incongruent with recent nutrition literature causing confusion among practitioners.

The **ASPEN Malnutrition Consensus Statement** from the Academy of Nutrition and Dietetics (Academy) and the American Society for Parenteral and Enteral Nutrition (ASPEN) has become a widely-adopted nutritional diagnostic standard in the U.S. since its publication in 2012.

ASPEN defines malnutrition as undernutrition meaning any nutrition imbalance.

ASPEN CRITERIA

The ASPEN diagnosis of malnutrition is based on the presence of at least **two of six characteristics** distinguishing non-severe and severe malnutrition in three different clinical contexts:

1. **Acute illness** or injury (duration of < 3 months) such as GI surgery, multi-system trauma, intubation, prolonged vomiting, or limited oral food intake.

2. **Chronic illness** (duration of 3 months or more) such as widespread metastatic cancer, severe malabsorption syndromes, HIV, or chemotherapy.

3. **Social/environmental** circumstances such as severe debilitation, the elderly living alone without social support, or lack of care.

ASPEN: Non-Severe (Moderate) Malnutrition (2 or more required)

Clinical Characteristics	Acute Context	Chronic Illness
Energy intake	< 75% estimated energy requirement for > 7 days	< 75% estimated energy requirement for ≥ 1 month
Weight loss (% of body weight)	1-2% in 1 week 5% in 1 month 7.5% in 3 months	5% in 1 month 7.5% in 3 months 10% in 6 months 20% in 1 year
Body fat loss	Mild	Mild
Muscle mass loss	Mild	Mild
Edema masking weight loss	Mild	Mild
Reduced grip strength	N/A	N/A

ASPEN: Severe Malnutrition (2 or more required)

Clinical Characteristics	Acute Context	Chronic Illness
Energy intake	< 50% estimated energy requirement for ≥ 5 days	< 75% estimated energy requirement for ≥ 1 month
Weight loss (% of body weight)	> 2% in 1 week > 5% in 1 month > 7.5% in 3 months	> 5% in 1 month > 7.5% in 3 months > 10% in 6 months > 20% in 1 year
Body fat loss	Moderate	Severe
Muscle mass loss	Moderate	Severe
Edema masking weight loss	Moderate to severe	Severe
Reduced grip strength	Measurably reduced	Measurably reduced

Notes:

- Weight loss and Edema should be considered mutually exclusive. To apply the edema characteristic, it must "mask weight loss;" therefore, if the weight loss criterion is met, it can't be "masked" by edema.
- Criteria for Social/Environmental context is the same as Chronic Illness except for energy intake for non-severe is < 75% estimated energy requirement for ≥ 3 months and for severe it is ≤ 50% estimated energy requirement for ≥ 1 month.

Some of the limitations of ASPEN have been that many criteria require subjective interpretation, the criteria are unfamiliar to providers, and the device to measure hand-grip strength is not widely available. There has also been some regulatory vulnerability with over-diagnosis of severe malnutrition.

Global Leadership Initiative on Malnutrition (GLIM) Definition: "GLIM Criteria for the Diagnosis of Malnutrition: A Consensus Report from the Global Clinical Nutrition Community" (January 2019) defines "malnutrition as a combination of reduced food intake or assimilation and varying degrees of acute or chronic inflammation, leading to altered body composition and diminished biological function." In other words, reduced calorie intake and increased calorie consumption causing adverse health consequences.

GLIM has been endorsed by all major nutrition societies world-wide including the American Society of Parenteral and Enteral Nutrition and the Academy of Nutrition and Dietetics.

GLIM Criteria. GLIM requires at least one of three phenotypic (clinical findings) criteria and one of two etiologic (causes) criteria. Severity of malnutrition is based on phenotypic criteria only.

Phenotypic Criteria	Non-Severe Criteria	Severe Criteria
Weight loss % (unintended)	5% ≤ 6 months, or 10% > 6 months	> 10% ≤ 6 months, or > 20% > 6 months
Low BMI	< 20 if < 70 yrs, or < 22 if ≥ 70 yrs	< 18.5 if < 70 yrs, or < 20 if ≥ 70 yrs
Reduced Muscle Mass	Reduced by objective measures and/or physical exam	Severe Deficit
Etiologic Criteria		
Reduced Nutritional Intake	< 50% of requirement > 1 week, or any reduction > 2 weeks, or chronic GI disorders with adverse nutrition impact	Same as Non-Severe
Inflammation	Chronic disease, or acute disease/injury with severe systemic inflammation, or socioeconomic/ environmental starvation	Same as Non-Severe

To measure **muscle mass**, GLIM recommends use of DEXA, bio-electrical impedance analysis (BIA), ultrasound, CT or MRI, but these are costly and impractical. As an alternative, calf or arm circumference, physical exam and calibrated hand-grip strength may be used.

CT scan at the L-3 level has been shown to accurately predict loss of muscle mass and correlate with severity. Calf circumference (adjusted for BMI) has been shown to correlate with muscle mass.

C-reactive protein (CRP) is recommended to confirm chronic or severe **systemic inflammation**. Albumin/prealbumin and SIRS criteria may also be used but are unnecessary if CRP (reference range = 0.3-1.0) is elevated.

The GLIM **BMI criteria** may at first seem overstated since the CDC definition of "normal" in the general healthy population is 18.5 to 24.9. However, world-wide nutritional research has validated the contribution of GLIM BMI ranges to malnutrition and confirmed their adverse health consequences in acutely and chronically ill hospitalized patients.

TREATMENT

Non-severe malnutrition may be treated with simple modalities: nutrition counseling, nutritious diet, 1-2 daily liquid supplements (e.g., Boost). **Severe** malnutrition would need an aggressive approach such as a supervised nutritional diet, daily calorie counts, at least 2-3 daily liquid supplements, appetite stimulants (Megestrol), frequent follow-up with a nutritionist, enteral or total parenteral nutrition (TPN). TPN would only be used in very severe malnutrition or perhaps active severe GI disorders that make oral or enteral feeding impossible.

Keep in mind that enteral nutrition (G-tube or nasogastric feeding tube) is not used exclusively for malnutrition. Some other conditions include severe dysphagia, frequent aspiration, severe debilitating dementia, esophageal motility disorders, esophageal obstruction. Minimal or no treatment may be recommended for severe malnutrition in hospice patients near the end of life. A nutritionist and provider statement to this effect is valuable documentation in this situation.

CODING AND DOCUMENTATION CHALLENGES

Under-recognition and under treatment of malnutrition, sometimes even when severe, is widespread – truly a malnutrition crisis especially for the acutely ill. The need for provider education and awareness is great.

GLIM is intended to be a simple, clinically intuitive tool for provider use that will enhance recognition and diagnosis of malnutrition. It was not intended to replace ASPEN for nutritionists in the U.S., so both can be considered authoritative.

The diagnosis of malnutrition and its severity should not be made by checking-off a minimum number of criteria from a list. Each patient's unique and the overall clinical picture must be considered together with these criteria using good clinical judgment following a comprehensive nutrition assessment.

Mild, moderate, and unspecified malnutrition (E44.1, E44.0, E46) are classified as CCs, and severe malnutrition (E43) is an MCC. All are included in CMS-HCC 21. Codes E40 (kwashiorkor), E41 (nutritional marasmus) and E42 (marasmic kwashiorkor) are reserved for malnutrition specifically related to these conditions, are extremely rare in the United States, and should be infrequently coded.

Coding Clinic 2020 First Quarter addresses **provider countersignature** of the nutritionist assessment: "Your hospital may develop a facility-based policy to address whether documentation that is signed-off by the patient's provider is allowed to be used for coding purposes."

Emaciation is a clinical description of a patient who appears severely malnourished. It is now indexed to code E43, severe malnutrition. Coding Clinic 2017 Third Quarter states that code R64 (cachexia) should be used for emaciation that is not due to malnutrition.

Cancer cachexia (R64) is characterized by muscle mass loss without proportional loss of fat tissue primarily due to "hypermetabolism" (increased energy consumption) and inflammation with or without malnutrition. Weight loss is always severe. If malnutrition is a component, it is typically severe and a query may be warranted.

Sarcopenia (M62.84) is a condition characterized by muscle mass loss without proportional loss of fat tissue typically associated with severe malnutrition, so a query for malnutrition and severity is almost always warranted.

Clinical validation is critically important, especially for severe malnutrition. The OIG and Department of Justice have made large monetary recoveries from many hospitals and healthcare systems over the past decade based on a high number of claims with a diagnosis of severe malnutrition. In 2020 the OIG claimed that Medicare had been overbilled $1 billion for severe malnutrition and has recommended widespread audits to recover these reimbursements.

To ensure correct compliant coding and clinical validation of severe malnutrition, use caution when strictly applying the ASPEN criteria, particularly in the acute context. GLIM seems more consistent with the traditional concepts of malnutrition and perhaps easier to defend. It is also important that treatment is congruent with severe malnutrition.

References

- GLIM Criteria for the Diagnosis of Malnutrition: A Consensus Report From the Global Clinical Nutrition Community. J Parenter Enteral Nutr. 2019
- Academy/ASPEN Adult Malnutrition Consensus 2012: J Acad Nutr Diet 2012; 112: 730–738
- Jensen et al. Malnutrition Syndromes: A Conundrum vs Continuum. J Parenter Enteral Nutr 2009; 33(6):710–716
- UpToDate: Geriatric Nutrition: Nutritional Issues in older adults
- Measuring calf circumference: a practical tool to predict skeletal muscle mass via adjustment with BMI. American Journal of Clinical Nutrition 2021; 113: 1398–1399
- Muscle mass, assessed at diagnosis by L3-CT scan as a prognostic marker of clinical outcomes in patients with gastric cancer: A systematic review and meta-analysis. Clin Nutr 2020; 39: 2045-2054
- Coding Clinic 2020 First Quarter p. 4
- The Solution to Severe Malnutrition Denials: Document the Treatment! Pinsonandtang.com/resources

DEFINITION

ASPEN defines pediatric malnutrition as "an imbalance between nutrient requirements and intake that results in cumulative deficits of energy, protein, or micronutrients that may negatively affect growth, development, and other relevant outcomes."

DIAGNOSTIC CRITERIA

Defining pediatric malnutrition and its severity is complex and highly subjective with multiple criteria and definitions. The most authoritative references come from CDC, WHO, ASPEN, and the American Academy of Pediatrics. CDC/WHO applies specifically to age < 5 and only by inference for ages 5 and above. ASPEN claims validity for ages up to 20.

ASPEN points out that pediatric malnutrition is highly subjective based on clinical judgment considering five basic parameters:

1. Anthropomorphic (physical characteristics)—objective criteria
   - Age < 2 years use WHO growth charts
   - Age > 2 years use CDC growth charts
2. Cause of nutritional deficiency (illness vs. social/environmental)
3. Inflammatory state (SIRS)—present/not present
4. Pathogenic (disease) mechanism—such as cancer or malabsorption
5. Clinical manifestations—such as tissue wasting, developmental delay, delayed wound healing

Severity may be clinically judged by findings in the above five parameters. Objective criteria for malnutrition are measures like the WHO and CDC growth charts:

Severity	Weight for Age	Weight for Height	Height for Age
Mild	N/A	80–89%	90–94%
Moderate	60–80%	70–79%	85–89%
Severe	< 60%	< 70%	< 85%

Source: CDC/WTF: Measuring and Interpreting Malnutrition and Mortality.

These are not percentile scores but rather the percent of average for weight and height for age. The average is defined as the 50th percentile for age identified on the growth chart, divided by the child's actual weight or height to calculate the percent, and then compared with the table above.

> **EXAMPLE** A 10-year-old boy appears to have clinical evidence of malnutrition. His weight is 53 pounds. Referring to the CDC weight-for-age chart, the average weight (50th percentile) of 10-year-old boys is 70 pounds. Dividing 53 by 70 = 74% (indicator of moderate malnutrition).

BMI Z-scores, calculated using height and weight for children (>2–20 years), are also used as a screening tool to identify possible weight problems in children.

Calculating an accurate BMI Z-score or CDC/WHO growth measure can be challenging since these are dependent on accurate weight and height/length measurements which may not be current or available in the medical record.

Other factors to consider when identifying malnutrition in children are the nutritionist physical exam, nutritional intake, weight loss, falling growth curve, not meeting expected weight gains, and correcting for prematurity.

TREATMENT

Essentially same as adult.

References
- Consensus Statement of the Academy of Nutrition and Dietetics/American Society for Parenteral and Enteral Nutrition: Indicators recommended for the identification and documentation of pediatric malnutrition (undernutrition)
- WHO/CDC: Growth Charts: www.cdc.gov

DEFINITION

Mechanical ventilation is an invasive respiratory procedure that supports a patient's breathing, moving air (usually supplemented with oxygen and/or aerosolized medications) into and out of the lungs. The ventilator is connected to the patient's airways by an endotracheal (ETT) or tracheostomy tube.

Do not assign a code below unless the ventilator support is "invasive," i.e., delivered through an ETT or a tracheostomy. The root operation is "Performance."

- 5A1935Z: Respiratory ventilation < 24 consecutive hours
- 5A1945Z: Respiratory ventilation 24–96 consecutive hours
- 5A1955Z: Respiratory ventilation > 96 consecutive hours

Coding Clinic 2014 Fourth Quarter states that other continuous invasive ventilation support (BiPAP and CPAP) delivered via ETT or tracheostomy constitutes mechanical ventilation using the above codes. Although BiPAP and CPAP are often used to treat acute respiratory failure, they are not usually included in the above codes since they are not typically delivered via ETT or tracheostomy.

TO CALCULATE DURATION OF MECHANICAL VENTILATION:

Start time begins with the time of:

1. Endotracheal intubation (and subsequent initiation of mechanical ventilation)
2. Initiation of mechanical ventilation through a tracheostomy
3. Arrival time of a previously intubated patient or a patient with a tracheostomy who is already on mechanical ventilation.

Considered part of the initial (continuous) duration:

1. Removal and immediate replacement of endotracheal tubes including immediate re-intubation following self-extubation.
2. Change from endotracheal intubation to a tracheostomy (mechanical ventilation is continued).

3. Weaning of a patient is included in counting the initial (continuous) duration. There may be several attempts to wean the patient prior to extubation, and there may be times when the ventilator is not in use even though the patient is still intubated.

Duration ends with:

1. Endotracheal extubation (the patient may be disconnected from the ventilator, but duration continues until the patient is extubated)
2. Cessation of the ventilator support for patients with a tracheostomy (termination of ventilator dependency)
3. Discharge/transfer time while still on the ventilator

The patient may require a subsequent period(s) of mechanical ventilation during the same hospitalization, interrupted by a ventilator-free period(s). In this case, two (or more) separate respiratory ventilation codes would be reported, each according to the duration of that particular period of continuous mechanical ventilation.

Postoperative mechanical ventilation. Coding Clinic states that a code for mechanical ventilation (and intubation) should not be assigned postoperatively for mechanical ventilation that is considered a normal part of surgery. If the patient remains on mechanical ventilation for an extended period (several days) post surgery, the mechanical ventilation should be coded.

The general assumption is made that "*several days*," meaning 48 hours, would always be considered longer than normally expected. Begin counting from the time of intubation in the OR, but do not code the endotracheal intubation.

Following many procedures, post-operative mechanical ventilation is not normal or expected. For others only a brief period of mechanical ventilation (perhaps 12–24 hours) is the norm. It would be expected that some underlying problem (not the surgery itself) would have caused or prolonged the duration of mechanical ventilation. These circumstances should be clearly documented as unusual, what the cause was, and why less than 48 hours is not "normal" or expected for the type of surgery performed.

This situation rarely impacts DRG assignment since it will be driven by the surgical procedure. This Coding Clinic advice relates specifically to the assignment of mechanical ventilation codes postoperatively, not the diagnosis of respiratory failure.

Intubation for airway protection. Patients with a severely altered level of consciousness may have lost their "gag" reflex that helps protect the airway from aspiration of regurgitated stomach contents or upper airway accumulation of blood or secretions and are intubated and ventilated for "airway protection." Familiar clinical situations are head trauma, CVA, brain hemorrhage and drug overdose.

Some of these patients may be able to maintain pulmonary ventilation and acceptable blood gases without ventilation support, but require intubation and mechanical ventilation for "airway protection" only. See also ***Respiratory Failure***.

Mechanical ventilation using home equipment. Per Coding Clinic 2018 First Quarter, it is appropriate to code mechanical ventilation for those patients who are admitted to the hospital on a home ventilator since the patient is receiving ventilator assistance and being evaluated and monitored.

References

- Coding Clinic 2014 Fourth Quarter p. 3 and 11
- Coding Clinic 2018 First Quarter p. 13.

DEFINITION

Myocardial injury is a new term introduced by the Fourth Universal Definition of Myocardial Infarction (2018). It is defined as an elevation of cardiac troponin values with at least one value above the 99th percentile upper reference limit (URL), often identified as a "critical value."

Myocardial injury is considered **acute** when there is a rise and/or fall of troponin values, with at least one above the 99th percentile. When chronic, the troponin levels remain stable at a constantly elevated level. Myocardial injury may be due to ischemic or nonischemic causes, and acute or chronic.

Acute myocardial injury without evidence of acute myocardial ischemia (defined below) is not myocardial infarction. Non-MI troponin elevations, or "non-ischemic myocardial injury," can be due to non-ischemic causes such as heart failure, myocarditis, cardiomyopathy, catheter ablation, defibrillation, cardiac contusion, sepsis, CVA/hemorrhage, pulmonary embolism or hypertension, chemotherapy, and amyloidosis or sarcoidosis.

Myocardial ischemia is inadequate oxygen supply to the myocardium without damage to myocardial cells. The most common cause of ischemia is coronary artery disease (CAD). Patients who have CAD have chronically reduced oxygen supply to the myocardium putting them at risk for acute ischemia when oxygen demand exceeds oxygen supply.

Acute myocardial ischemia is evidenced by symptoms, EKG changes or positive cardiac imaging (see Diagnostic Criteria that follows). If troponin is also released and above the 99th percentile (i.e., acute myocardial injury), a myocardial infarction has occurred. If not, then the patient only has unstable angina or demand ischemia.

Myocardial infarction is irreversible ischemic damage or "injury" to the myocardium. An acute myocardial infarction occurs when acute myocardial ischemia causes acute myocardial injury.

The diagnosis of myocardial ischemia involves the physician's clinical judgment of the patient's clinical circumstances.

Types of MI
- Type 1: Coronary artery disease with plaque rupture and coronary thrombosis (STEMI and NSTEMI)
- Type 2: Imbalance between oxygen supply and myocardial demand without thrombosis
- Type 3: Myocardial infarction resulting in death when biomarker values are unavailable
- Type 4a: Myocardial infarction related to percutaneous coronary intervention (PCI)
- Type 4b: Myocardial infarction related to stent thrombosis
- Type 4c: Myocardial infarction due to restenosis ≥50% after an initially successful PCI
- Type 5: Myocardial infarction related to CABG

Type 1 STEMI is due to CAD and is usually self-evident with characteristic EKG findings and typically requires immediate reperfusion therapy or percutaneous coronary intervention (PCI). **NSTEMI** is also due to CAD and identified by elevated troponin but may have only minor non-specific ST/T-wave changes or even a normal EKG.

Type 2 MI is recognized by elevated troponin not due to CAD and primarily due to supply/demand imbalance. Common causes include coronary artery spasm or embolism, atrial fibrillation, sustained tachyarrhythmia, severe bradycardia, severe anemia, hypotension, shock, or severe hypertension.

Unstable angina and **demand ischemia** are defined by symptoms consistent with acute myocardial ischemia, but without acute myocardial injury (elevated troponins > 99th percentile). The difference between the two diagnoses is that unstable angina is due to CAD and demand ischemia is not.

Acute coronary syndrome (ACS) encompasses symptoms consistent with myocardial ischemia due to CAD but is only a provisional diagnosis until a more specific diagnosis can be made after evaluation (e.g., NSTEMI, unstable angina, other cardiac or non-cardiac cause).

DIAGNOSTIC CRITERIA

Type I MI (STEMI & NSTEMI) criteria include acute myocardial injury and evidence of acute myocardial ischemia due to CAD. Evidence of **acute myocardial ischemia** includes at least one of the following:

1. Symptoms of acute myocardial ischemia: Chest pain (pressure, heaviness, tightness or constriction), neck, jaw, shoulder or arm pain; shortness of breath; nausea, vomiting; sweating, profound fatigue or weakness; syncope, presyncope, palpitations. However, some people (especially diabetics and the elderly) experience only minimal symptoms or no symptoms at all making the physician's clinical judgment essential.

2. New ischemic EKG changes: Non-specific STT changes, non-specific changes, ST-depression, new LBBB, T-wave inversion. STEMI: ST-elevation [in specific leads], or acute MI [anterior, lateral, inferior, posterior, septal, anterolateral, anteroseptal.

3. Imaging evidence:
   - Echocardiogram: Regional or global wall motion abnormalities, new systolic or diastolic dysfunction
   - Radionuclide imaging (myocardial perfusion imaging, SPECT): Regional wall motional abnormalities (anterior, inferior, posterior), extent of infarction, LV function (reduced ejection fraction)
   - MRI heart and CT coronary angiogram: Myocardial structure, function and perfusion, affected coronary arteries
   - Cardiac cath and angiogram: identification of a coronary clot or thrombus (STEMI)

Note that cardiac stress tests can be conducted using EKG only, echocardiogram, or radionuclide imaging. The patient may be "stressed" by walking on a treadmill or, if unable, by medication-induced tachycardia with dipyridamole (Persantine), adenosine, or dobutamine. Radionuclide imaging is most commonly used.

"**Silent**" (asymptomatic) myocardial ischemia is defined as the presence of objective evidence of myocardial ischemia (ischemic changes on EKG, positive cardiac imaging) in the absence of chest discomfort or other anginal symptoms, e.g., dyspnea, nausea, diaphoresis, etc.

Type 2 MI criteria include acute myocardial injury (elevated troponin > 99th percentile URL) with evidence of acute myocardial ischemia (see above) that is not due to CAD. Ischemia is due to myocardial oxygen demand that exceeds myocardial oxygen supply (supply-demand mismatch).

TREATMENT

Type 1 STEMI usually requires immediate reperfusion therapy such as coronary stent (PCI) or fibrinolysis, CABG, antithrombotic or heparin-like drugs, beta-blocker, ACEI.

Type 1 NSTEMI may be treated with nitroglycerin, aspirin,beta-blocker, ACEI, heparin-like drug, antithrombotic, e.g., Plavix, Aggrastat.

Type 2 MI treatment is directed at correcting the underlying cause, such severe anemia, atrial fibrillation, sustained tachyarrhythmia, severe bradycardia, hypotension, shock, or severe hypertension. A cardiac workup (stress, echo) may be ordered to rule out an ischemic cause.

Management of Type 4b and 4c is similar to Type 1. Treatment of Types 4a and 5 depends on the associated circumstances, but thrombolytics and anti-thrombotics may be hazardous in the setting of PCI and CABG. PCI may be employed.

CODING AND DOCUMENTATION CHALLENGES

The clinical validity of acute myocardial infarction requires both (1) acute myocardial injury, and (2) evidence of acute myocardial ischemia based on the definitions above.

As of October 1, 2021, there is a new code, I5A, for non-ischemic myocardial injury [non-traumatic] which is a CC. Non-ischemic myocardial injury is: (1) elevated troponins above the 99th percentile (myocardial injury), (2) lack of evidence of acute myocardial ischemia (defined above), and (3) the elevated troponins are not due to CAD, but due to non-ischemic causes such as heart failure, myocarditis, cardiomyopathy, etc. To assign I5A, a diagnosis of myocardial injury or non-ischemic myocardial injury would also need to be documented.

> **EXAMPLE** Patient admitted with pulmonary embolism and respiratory failure and elevated troponins > 99th percentile that trended down. Patient has no symptoms and echo shows no wall motion abnormalities. Physician diagnosis: "Elevated troponins due to PE." Should I query for Type 2 MI?

In the above case example, this would not be a Type 2 MI. Although there was acute myocardial injury (elevated troponins with rise and/or fall), there was no evidence of acute myocardial ischemia, and the physician documented the elevated troponins were due to the PE. The elevated troponins due to PE would be considered a "non-MI" or "non-ischemic" cause of the myocardial injury. A query for non-ischemic myocardial injury would be appropriate in this case.

Troponin levels. For different labs, the reference ranges vary. Troponin I is preferred to troponin T. In general, higher troponin levels are associated with more extensive myocardial injury. Peak troponin values are usually highest with STEMI, then NSTEMI, and lowest overall in non-ischemic (non-MI) causes. Keep in mind though that very high troponin levels alone are not diagnostic of a myocardial infarction and must be supported by evidence of acute myocardial ischemia.

The term "demand ischemia" may be used indiscriminately for supply/demand circumstances even when patients experience acute myocardial injury (elevated troponins) indicative of Type 2 MI.

Always query regarding the possibility of NSTEMI or Type 2 MI when the diagnosis of ACS, unstable angina, or demand ischemia is associated with elevated troponins and meets the diagnostic criteria above.

NSTEMI should be reserved for MI due to CAD, and Type 2 MI should be used for MI not due to CAD. Otherwise, the MI will be misclassified.

Acute MI documented as due to demand ischemia or ischemic imbalance or as Type 2 NSTEMI or STEMI, should be assigned to code I21. A1, **Type 2 MI** (see the ICD-10 classification, OCG section I.C.9.e.5, and Coding Clinic, Fourth Quarter, page 12). A Type 2 MI cannot be assigned as principal diagnosis. Code first the underlying cause, such as anemia, COPD, paroxysmal tachycardia, shock.

If a NSTEMI evolves to STEMI, assign the STEMI code. If a STEMI converts to NSTEMI due to thrombolytic therapy, it is still coded as STEMI.

STEMI codes have specificity options for the involved site (wall) and the involved artery. If the site or artery is not specified, this information can be gleaned from other sources in the medical record such as an EKG or cath report.

Initial vs. subsequent MI. An MI is classified as acute for the 4 weeks following its occurrence. If another MI occurs within that 4-week period, it is identified as a subsequent MI and two codes must be assigned.

- Initial MI (I21.-) is assigned when the patient is admitted for the initial episode of care, or for an MI that occurred within the past 4 weeks—but only if it meets the OCG definition for "other diagnoses". If another MI occurs more than 4 weeks after a prior MI, it is coded as an initial MI, not subsequent.

- Subsequent MI (I22.-) is assigned when the patient is admitted with another MI within 4 weeks of an initial MI. An initial MI code (describing the site of the initial MI) must also be assigned whenever a subsequent MI occurs. Sequencing of these codes depends on the circumstances of admission.

Subsequent MI codes apply only to Type 1 STEMI and NSTEMI, not Type 2 MI (I21A1) or other types. Old MI (I25.2) is used for a healed MI > 4 weeks old or past MI but currently presenting no symptoms.

For **DRG Tips,** see DRGs 280-282, Acute myocardial infarction, discharged alive.

References

- The Fourth Universal Definition of Myocardial Infarction (2018)

- 2011 ACCF/AHA Focused Update of the Guidelines for the Management of Patients with Unstable Angina/Non–ST-Elevation Myocardial Infarction, J Am Coll Cardiol 2011;57: 1920–1959

- 2014 AHA/ACC Guideline for the Management of Patients With Non–ST-Elevation Acute Coronary Syndromes. J Am Coll Cardiol; 64: e139– 228

- ACC/AHA 2007 Guidelines for the Management of Patients With Unstable Angina/Non ST-Elevation Myocardial Infarction, Circulation 2007;116: e148-e304

- UpToDate.com: Silent myocardial ischemia: Epidemiology, diagnosis, treatment, and prognosis

- Coding Clinic 2019 Second Quarter p. 5

- Coding Clinic 2017 Fourth Quarter p. 12

- Coding Clinic 2013 First Quarter p. 25

- Coding Clinic 2012 Fourth Quarter p. 102.

DEFINITION

Abnormal, uncontrolled cell growth resulting in tumor formation. Benign remains localized; some benign neoplasms can be fatal when vital structures are intricately involved. Malignant (cancer) is capable of metastasis (non-contiguous spread to distant sites).

- Primary site = origin of the cancer
- Secondary sites = metastatic, or extension or invasion into other sites

TREATMENT OF MALIGNANT NEOPLASMS

Most commonly treated by surgical removal, chemotherapy, and radiation therapy. Others include bone marrow transplant, stem cell transplant, cryotherapy, brachytherapy, immunotherapy, hyperthermia, laser, angiogenesis inhibitors.

CODING AND DOCUMENTATION CHALLENGES

Coding rules assign codes for secondary (metastatic) sites according to the affected metastatic site. For example, primary breast cancer with metastasis to the vertebra is coded as primary site = breast, secondary (metastatic) site = vertebra. Clinically this secondary site would be described as metastatic breast cancer.

If the primary neoplasm has been eradicated (e.g., surgical removal, stem cell transplant) and there is no further treatment, it is coded as "history of" the primary malignancy (category Z85) to identify the origin of the neoplasm. Residual metastases are coded as secondary sites.

When a primary neoplasm has been eradicated but is still being treated (chemotherapy, radiation, etc.), the primary neoplasm should still be coded. The principal diagnosis will depend upon the circumstances of the admission.

When a patient is admitted because of metastatic cancer and the treatment is directed toward the metastasis, the metastasis should be the principal diagnosis even if the primary malignancy is still present. For example, patient with metastatic lung cancer admitted for altered mental status due to brain metastases.

Contiguous sites. Extension, invasion, or metastasis to another site (organ) is coded as a secondary malignant neoplasm. Use only a single primary neoplasm code when two or more contiguous sites within the *same organ* overlap (use subcategory .8 overlapping lesion if point of origin unknown). Use multiple primary neoplasm codes for multiple sites in the same organ that do not overlap (e.g., tumors in different quadrants of the same breast). See OCG I.C.2.

EXAMPLES Thyroid cancer with extension into the trachea, would be coded to primary thyroid cancer (C73) with secondary malignancy of trachea (C78.39).

Malignant neoplasm of the transverse colon invading the duodenum would be coded C18.4 (primary neoplasm of transverse colon) and C78.4 (secondary neoplasm of small intestine).

Adenocarcinoma of the duodenum and jejunum would be coded to C17.8 (malignant neoplasm of overlapping sites of small intestine).

Carcinoma of the tip of the tongue extending to involve the ventral surface is coded to C02.1 (malignant neoplasm border/tip of tongue) as the point of origin is known.

Complications. When the reason for admission is *only* treatment of a complication, such as dehydration, associated with the neoplasm or adverse effects of chemotherapy/radiotherapy, and the complication is the focus of treatment (not the malignancy), sequence the complication or adverse effect as principal diagnosis.

An exception to this rule is an admission for management of **anemia** associated with the malignancy. Even if the treatment is only for anemia, the malignancy is sequenced as the principal diagnosis. On the other hand, if any treatment or evaluation is directed toward the primary or secondary neoplasm, the neoplasm should be the principal diagnosis. Note this does not apply to pancytopenia or neutropenia.

Principal diagnosis. Always review the record to determine if the malignancy can be assigned as the principal diagnosis rather than a complication or another condition. Patients are often admitted with numerous complications that, after study, are ultimately found to be related to or due to the patient's malignancy. Review the circumstances of admission, workup, evaluation or treatment (or decision not to treat or patient goes to hospice or expires) to support the malignancy as principal diagnosis.

Signs and symptoms associated with an existing primary or secondary neoplasm cannot be used to replace the neoplasm as principal diagnosis, regardless of the number of admissions or encounters for treatment and care of the neoplasm.

Admission for radio-/immuno-/chemo-therapy. If the patient is admitted solely for the purpose of receiving external beam radiotherapy, chemotherapy or immunotherapy, code Z51.0, Z51.11, or Z51.12 is sequenced as principal diagnosis. If one of these was not the sole reason for the admission but was also for workup, staging, or other treatment of cancer, the malignancy could be sequenced as the principal diagnosis.

If a patient admission is for the insertion or implantation of radio-active elements (e.g., brachytherapy), the appropriate code for the malignancy is sequenced as the principal or first-listed diagnosis. Code Z51.0 should not be assigned.

Common comorbidities associated with malignancy include metastases, pancytopenia, malnutrition, BMI < 20, cerebral (brain) edema or compression, respiratory failure, depression, encephalopathy, coma, sepsis, aspiration pneumonia, AKI/ATN, pathologic fracture.

Pathology reports. According to Coding Clinic, for inpatient cases it is not appropriate to code a diagnosis directly from the pathology report since a pathologist's interpretation is not the same as a diagnosis provided by a physician directly involved in the care and treatment of the patient. For example, if the attending physician documented "brain mass" and the pathologist documented "meningioma," this would require clarification from the attending physician. Note that this is different for outpatients.

Post-discharge pathology reports. Some providers may be reluctant to document the clinical significance (diagnosis) of a pathology report that was unavailable prior to discharge and mistakenly believe that entering a diagnosis in the record post-discharge is somehow improper.

Quite to the contrary, it is very important to make a currently dated addendum to the record acknowledging post-discharge findings and documenting patient notification and arrangements for necessary follow-up. Failure to do so may expose both the provider and the hospital to potential claims of medical negligence.

Queries for post-discharge documentation should be addressed to the provider who requested the test or performed the procedure resulting in the report, since this is the person who is legally accountable for notifying the patient and arranging follow-up.

Metastatic cancers are included in CMS-HCC 8 (Metastatic Cancer & Acute Leukemia) and is the highest-weight CMS-HCC.

References
- Official Coding Guidelines, Section I.C.2
- Coding Clinic 2016 Third Quarter p. 25: Coding from Pathology Report.

DEFINITION

Pancreatitis is inflammation of the pancreas not typically associated with infection. It can be acute or chronic; it may be mild or severe and even potentially life-threatening.

Causes include: Alcoholism, elevated triglycerides (especially with diabetes), hypercalcemia, medications, and gallstone obstruction of the pancreatic or common bile duct (gallstone pancreatitis).

Common bile duct obstruction or pancreatic duct obstruction is particularly serious and may progress to life-threatening ascending cholangitis or pancreatic abscess.

Acute pancreatitis. Symptoms are typically acute abdominal/back pain; often fever, elevated white blood cell count, non-infectious SIRS, vomiting. Complications include hypocalcemia, ileus, acute kidney injury, sepsis or ARDS. Pancreatic enzymes amylase and lipase are usually both elevated; lipase is the more sensitive test.

Acute pancreatitis may lead to chronic pancreatitis, pancreatic insufficiency, pseudocyst, or abscess. Mortality from acute pancreatitis ranges from 2–9% with higher risk if age >55, BMI >30, organ failure, or alcoholism.

Chronic pancreatitis. The usual manifestation of chronic pancreatitis is chronic abdominal pain requiring chronic opioid analgesics. Amylase may be normal but lipase is a more sensitive test and usually elevated. Recurrent acute exacerbations are characteristic which may require inpatient admission.

Chronic pancreatitis may result in pancreatic insufficiency requiring long-term oral enzyme replacement such as Creon, Pancrease, Viokase, Zenpep.

It can cause secondary diabetes due to destruction of insulin-producing pancreatic islet cells. In up to 10% of cases, patients may develop pancreatic pseudocyst or pancreatic cancer (the 20-year risk is 5%).

DIAGNOSTIC CRITERIA FOR ACUTE PANCREATITIS

The American College of Gastroenterology recommends that **two or more** of the following three findings would usually indicate acute pancreatitis:

- Abdominal pain consistent with pancreatitis
- Lipase and/or amylase > 3 times upper reference limit
- Characteristic findings on imaging studies (ultrasound, CT, MRI)

Pain associated with pancreatitis is typically severe, constant, steady, boring in nature—not dull, colicky, or of varying intensity. Location is usually LUQ, left flank, back or epigastric. Elevation of amylase and lipase < 3 times upper reference limit is nonspecific and can be caused by many conditions such as gastroenteritis, cholecystitis, bowel obstruction, peptic ulcer.

TREATMENT

Acute pancreatitis: May include IV pain medication, IV fluid resuscitation, NPO/NG-suction; sometimes IV antibiotics (if infection is suspected). Ultrasound is usually performed for evaluation and to rule out biliary/pancreatic obstruction.

Contrast-enhanced CT or MRI is usually reserved for uncertain or refractory cases. Diagnostic/therapeutic endoscopy is usually employed including retrograde cholangio-pancreatography (ERCP). If necessary, removal of an obstructing common duct stone can be done endoscopically.

Chronic pancreatitis: Chronic abdominal pain usually requires chronic opioid analgesics. If it results in pancreatic insufficiency, long-term oral enzyme replacement such as Creon, Pancrease, Viokase, Zenpep may be required.

Pancreatic cyst or pseudocyst may require drainage if it is large (greater than 6–12 cm) or if symptomatic or complicated by infection, abscess, fistula, ascites, or biliary obstruction.

CODING AND DOCUMENTATION CHALLENGES

When a patient has acute pancreatitis or acute exacerbation of chronic pancreatitis, it is usually the principal diagnosis, but the codes are also MCCs. It should be distinguished from chronic pancreatitis.

ICD-10 has multiple codes for acute pancreatitis, all of which are MCCs allowing greater specificity: idiopathic, biliary, alcoholic, drug-induced, and other.

The 5th character identifies whether there is infected necrosis, necrosis without infection, or no infection or necrosis. There is no code for infection without necrosis, so in this case the only available code is "with infected necrosis" (perhaps presuming that infection always produces some necrosis).

Chronic pancreatitis (K86.1–a CC) is not usually the principal reason for admission unless there is an acute exacerbation (K85.90). Treatment, if continued as an inpatient, may include chronic opioid analgesics for pain and enzyme replacement if the patient has pancreatic insufficiency.

Recurrent or relapsing pancreatitis is coded as "chronic," but is likely to be an acute exacerbation if it is the reason for admission. A query might be needed for clarification.

References

- Management of Acute Pancreatitis. Am J Gastroenterol 2013; 108:1400–1415
- Cleveland Clinic: Acute Pancreatitis
- UpToDate.com: Clinical Manifestations and Diagnosis of Acute Pancreatitis.

DEFINITION

Pancytopenia is a simultaneous deficiency of all three blood cell lineages: red blood cells, platelets, and neutrophils. Its clinical significance is the triple impact of anemia (decreased tissue oxygen supply), thrombocytopenia (bleeding), and neutropenia (susceptibility to infection).

There are many possible causes including malignancy, chemotherapy, other medications, myelodysplasia, aplastic anemia, radiation, splenomegaly.

DIAGNOSTIC CRITERIA

- Neutropenia: Absolute neutrophils (ANC) < 1.8 k
- Thrombocytopenia: Platelets < 150 k
- Anemia: Hgb < 13.0 gm/dL (men), < 12.0 (women)

Neutropenia is an absolute neutrophil count (ANC) < 1.8 k which is the lower limit of the reference range. Severity of neutropenia can be classified as mild (1.0–1.5), moderate (0.5–1.0), and severe (< 0.5).

The ANC is almost always reported on a CBC in hospitalized patients. If the ANC is not available, WBC < 4,000 is a good proxy for ANC although it is not definitive. If the WBC is borderline or in the low normal range, an ANC should be obtained to determine the presence of neutropenia or can be calculated with WBC, neutrophils and bands.

Thrombocytopenia is a platelet count below the lower reference limit (<150 k). Severity can be classified as mild (100 to 150 k), moderate (50 to 99 k), and severe (< 50 k). The risk of bleeding is minimal until the thrombocytopenia is severe (< 50 k).

Anemia is defined by the World Health Organization as hemoglobin (Hgb) < 13 gm (men); < 12 gm (women), and < 11 gm (pregnancy).

TREATMENT

Treatment of pancytopenia is usually directed at the cause and/or correction of one or more of the three suppressed cell lines. Anemia and thrombocytopenia may be treated with transfusion. Sometimes epoetin alfa (Epogen, Procrit) is given for anemia. Granulocyte colony-stimulating factor (G-CSF) like filgrastim (Neupogen) is commonly used for severe neutropenia to stimulate bone marrow production.

CODING AND DOCUMENTATION CHALLENGES

Identification of chemotherapy or other drugs as the cause of pancytopenia is crucial since these codes are MCCs. Pancytopenia caused by chemotherapy is coded as D61.810, if caused by other drugs D61.811. Unspecified pancytopenia is coded to D61.818 which is a CC.

Pancytopenia is **not separately coded** with aplastic anemia, myelodysplasia, myeloproliferative disease, HIV disease/AIDS, and several other rare conditions. Pancytopenia can be coded with acute myeloid leukemia per Coding Clinic.

For patients who have neutropenia and anemia secondary to chemotherapy (D70.1, D64.81) and also have thrombocytopenia, a separate code can be assigned for thrombocytopenia (D69.59), but pancytopenia would not be coded. See Coding Clinic 2014 Fourth Quarter, p. 22.

References

- UpToDate.com: Approach to the adult with pancyopenia
- Pancytopenia. National Library of Medicine: Stat Pearls NBK563146
- Coding Clinic 2014 Fourth Quarter p. 22
- Coding Clinic 2019 First Quarter p. 16.

DEFINITION

Fracture in abnormal bone due to minor trauma (or occurring spontaneously) that would not be expected to cause a fracture in normal, healthy bone.

Osteoporosis is decreased bone density below a certain threshold measured by DEXA. Osteopenia is decreased bone density above the osteoporosis threshold measured by DEXA and a precursor of osteoporosis.

DIAGNOSTIC CRITERIA

- **Minor or no trauma.** Significant trauma is defined, among other things, as a fall from a height of six feet or more. Simply falling from a sitting or standing position or getting out of bed does not usually cause a fracture in normal bone, and represents only minor trauma.

- **Abnormal underlying bone.** Osteoporosis (most common cause), multiple myeloma, other neoplasms (malignant or benign), bone cyst, and osteogenesis imperfecta.

DEXA scanning is the usual diagnostic tool for osteoporosis. Osteoporosis cannot be detected on x-ray until it becomes severe.

TREATMENT

Treatment of acute pathological fractures includes pain management with opioid analgesics, NSAIDs, Tylenol, bracing, and physical therapy. Kyphoplasty for vertebral compression fractures is usually not necessary unless the patient remains incapacitated after at least several weeks of aggressive pain management.

Treatment of osteoporosis includes Fosamax, Boniva, Actonel, Reclast, Prolia, vitamin D, Forteo, Atelvia, Fortical, Miacalcin, Evista, calcium.

CODING AND DOCUMENTATION CHALLENGES

Official Coding Guidelines I.C.13.d.2: "A code from category M80 [Osteoporosis with current pathological fracture], not a traumatic fracture code, should be used for any patient with known osteoporosis who suffers a fracture, even if the patient had a minor fall or trauma, if that fall or trauma would not usually break a normal, healthy bone."

CDI and coding specialists should usually be able to make this determination without a query and encouraged to do so pursuant to the above OCG section; if uncertain, query the provider.

Most patients over age 60 who sustain fractures after minor trauma (like falling from a standing position) have **osteoporosis**.

X-ray cannot detect osteoporosis until it has become severe, and radiologists often use the term "**osteopenia**" ("poverty" of bone) to describe the x-ray appearance of severe osteoporosis. Neither clinical osteopenia nor mild to moderate osteoporosis can be seen on X-ray which is why DEXA scanning is used for diagnosis. Only severe osteoporosis can be seen on x-ray.

Terms classified as pathologic fractures include osteoporotic, fragility, neoplastic, non-traumatic, insufficiency, spontaneous, chronic.

As principal diagnosis (without a surgical procedure), pathologic fractures are assigned to DRGs 542–544, Pathologic fractures. They are CCs as a secondary diagnosis, except stress and fatigue fractures.

In most cases, the 7th character would be assigned as **A (initial treatment)** as long as the patient is undergoing active treatment for the fracture which is often only pain medications.

Lumbar compression fractures are classified as "traumatic" and assigned to back pain DRGs 551-552 which are frequently audited and denied for inpatient medical necessity. Pathologic fracture DRGs are nearly always medically necessary and rarely audited.

Pathologic fractures occurring during admission are excluded as Hospital Acquired Conditions (HAC).

References

- Journal of Neurosurgery: Trends in pathological vertebral fractures in the United States: 1993 to 2004
- University of Washington Department of Radiology: Fractures Without Significant Trauma
- UpToDate.com: Osteoporotic thoracolumbar vertebral compression fractures: Clinical manifestations and treatment
- UpToDate.com: Evaluation and management of complete and impending pathologic fractures in patients with metastatic bone disease, multiple myeloma, and lymphoma
- Official Coding Guidelines I.C.13.c and d.

DEFINITION

Pneumonia generally refers to lung infection. It is most commonly caused by viruses or bacteria, but other causes include fungi, parasites, aspiration, chemicals, toxins, or physical injury to the lungs.

The term pneumonitis generally refers clinically to an inflammatory reaction without implying causation.

DIAGNOSTIC CRITERIA

Pneumonia is a clinical diagnosis, not culture-based, and usually confirmed by chest x-ray.

- **Symptoms** may include fever, chills, cough, sputum, shortness of breath, pleuritic chest pain. Respiratory distress can progress to respiratory failure.

- **Physical exam** may show rales, rhonchi, bronchial breath sounds, dullness, pleural rub, chest wall splinting.

- **WBC** may be low, normal, or elevated.

- **Chest x-ray** usually shows consolidation, infiltrate or interstitial changes which may be delayed in appearance by one or two days, especially if the patient is initially dehydrated. There may be a pneumonic pleural effusion which may progress to empyema (pleural abscess).

- **CT scan** is more sensitive than chest x-ray and may occasionally demonstrate infiltrates or consolidation when chest x-ray does not.

- Blood and sputum **cultures** are usually negative, but when positive, guide more specific antibiotic selection.

Pneumonia may be diagnosed on **clinical grounds** alone even when imaging (X-ray, CT) is negative. To avoid confusion, the provider ought to make a specific reference to the clinical basis of the diagnosis also noting the absence of radiographic findings.

TREATMENT

The presumed (suspected) organism can be determined by the choice of antibiotics, considering the risk for multi-drug resistance. A full course of treatment lasting a total of 7–14 days would be expected to validate a diagnosis of pneumonia, although a high-dose short course (5 days) of Levaquin is approved for community-acquired pneumonia (CAP).

Antibiotic	Treatment for
Aztreonam, cefazoline, cefepime, cefotaxime, ceftazidime, ertapenem, meropenem, primaxin	Gram-negatives (especially Pseudomonas)
Ciprofloxacin	Pseudomonas; Hemophilus
Clindamycin	Aspiration; staph and strep; anaerobes
Doxycycline	Gram positive and Hemophilus; also Legionella
Flagyl (metronidazole)	Aspiration; anaerobes
Gentamycin, tobramycin, amikacin	Gram-negatives
Levaquin (levofloxacin), moxifloxacin, gemifloxacin	CAP; Aspiration
Oxacillin, dicloxacillin, flucloxacillin	Staph (MSSA)
Rocephin (ceftriaxone)	CAP
Vancomycin	Staph (MRSA)
Zithromax (azithromycin), clarithromycin	CAP
Zosyn	Gram-negatives (excl. Hemophilus); Aspiration
Zyvox	Vancomycin-resistant gram-positives incl. MRSA

The Infectious Disease Society of America and the American Thoracic Society (IDSA/ATS) have dropped the **HCAP pneumonia category** based on new research that it was overly sensitive, did not demonstrate as high a risk for multi-drug resistant organisms as previously thought, and lacked sufficient evidence of a significant impact on outcomes. Over-utilization of broad-spectrum antibiotics was another compelling consideration. It is recommended that patients who would have been previously classified as having HCAP should be managed in a way similar to those with CAP, deciding whether to include gram negative and MRSA treatment on a case-by-case basis.

Many providers continue to use the HCAP terminology, and if so it implies gram-negatives and/or staph as the most likely/suspected organisms if the antibiotics selected are consistent with it.

TYPES OF PNEUMONIA

Community Acquired Pneumonia (CAP) is acquired outside the hospital in the absence of MDR circumstances (see below). Viral is the most common cause of CAP, followed by Pneumococcus, Hemophilus, Chlamydia, or Mycoplasma.

Gram Negative Pneumonia. Pneumonia due to gram-negative organisms including E. coli, Klebsiella, Proteus, Serratia, Pseudomonas, Enterobacter, and others. Clinical indicators include elderly, debilitated, or nursing home resident; cancer, chemotherapy, COPD, or chronic illness and also high-risk MDR circumstances below.

Staphylococcal (MRSA/MSSA) Pneumonia. Clinical indicators include those with indwelling IV catheters/devices, G-tube, ESRD, open wounds/skin ulcers, recent antibiotic therapy (especially broad-spectrum), postoperative status, immune-suppressed, IV drug use, ventilator status, empyema.

For all infections, **antibiotic resistance** is the result of overuse of antibiotics and occurs when bacteria (or other microorganisms) have been exposed to different antibiotics over long periods of time and develop resistance to them. Multi-drug resistant (**MDR**) organisms demonstrate resistance to multiple antibiotics especially those used most often to treat infections. Well-known MDR bacteria include E. coli, Pseudomonas, other gram-negatives, MRSA, enterococcus.

Treatment of MDR infections typically requires one or more potent, broad-spectrum antibiotics like vancomycin, Zosyn, cefepime, Primaxin, etc., often for 14 days or more. See ***Antimicrobial Resistance.***

Consider a patient with a Pseudomonas infection and no MDR risk who may be treated with Cipro, but if any MDR risk factor, a drug like Primaxin might be needed. On the other hand, an otherwise healthy person with a lobar pneumonia who lives with and cares for someone with a chronic MRSA wound infection would need vancomycin pending gram stain and culture results.

Aspiration pneumonia occurs when food, saliva, liquids, or vomitus is aspirated into bronchi or lungs. Aspiration pneumonia is more common than generally believed and often overlooked. Clinical indicators suggesting aspiration are:

- RLL infiltrate on chest x-ray is "classic" location
- Residence in nursing facility; debilitated, bed-confined
- Esophageal disorder: obstruction, motility, stenosis, cancer
- Altered level of consciousness
- Alcoholism, severe intoxication, illicit drug use, overdose
- Recent vomiting; presence of NG tube
- Impaired gag reflex, dysphagia, gastroparesis or GERD
- History of CVA or neurodegenerative disorder
- Positive swallowing study is highly suggestive; a negative study does not rule out aspiration.

Hospital-Acquired Pneumonia (HAP) is clinically defined as pneumonia that occurs 48 hours or more after admission and was not incubating at the time of admission. Typically treated for gram-negatives and/or staph.

Ventilator-Associated Pneumonia (VAP) is defined as pneumonia that develops 48 hours or more after mechanical ventilation is initiated by means of an endotracheal tube or tracheostomy. VAP is usually hospital-acquired but can occur in patients who are chronically ventilator dependent. Causative organisms are usually Pseudomonas or staph (especially MRSA) and sometimes other gram-negatives.

Occasionally a patient requiring intubation may have aspirated before or during intubation and its appearance may be delayed for 1–2 days. This situation should be clarified to avoid misclassification as VAP.

CODING AND DOCUMENTATION CHALLENGES

Providers should always document their reasoning when pneumonia is diagnosed on clinical grounds alone without chest x-ray findings.

ICD-10 coding and DRG classification of pneumonia is based on causation (organisms, aspiration, radiation, etc.). To be assigned to the appropriate DRG, the provider must identify the probable, suspected, or definitive organism(s) or other cause of the pneumonia. "Simple pneumonia" is assigned to DRGs 193-195 and complex pneumonia to higher-weighted 177-178 "Respiratory Infections."

Positive sputum cultures cannot be used to assign a specific type of pneumonia without the provider's confirmation. The provider must state that the pneumonia is due to a particular organism. For example, "Klebsiella pneumonia," or "Pneumonia due to E. coli."

Whenever indicators of gram-negative or staph pneumonia are present and the patient is receiving IV antibiotics for gram-negatives or staph, the **likely or suspected organism** should be documented because such patients have higher costs and morbidity. For example, "Pneumonia likely due to staph."

IDSA/ATS recommend that gram-negative and/or staph antibiotics be discontinued if high-quality sputum gram stain and culture as well as blood cultures do not demonstrate any of those organisms. Obtaining a high-quality sputum specimen for gram stain and culture is more crucial than ever for effective guideline-based management.

Given the IDSA/ATS recommendations, it would be reasonable to assume that if the provider continues a full course (7-14 days) of gram negative and/or staph antibiotic therapy, these would be the most likely, suspected or presumed organisms causing pneumonia. If not documented as such, a query would be warranted citing the risk factors and antibiotic management.

For all infections, review for documentation of **antibiotic resistance** (Z16.10-Z16.39) in the culture results and progress notes. The provider must document an infection has become drug resistant, e.g., "multi-drug resistant" or "resistant to [specified drug]." If not, a query may be necessary. Do not assign a Z16 category code if the infection code identifies the drug resistance, e.g., MRSA pneumonia.

For patients with **COPD and pneumonia**, sequencing of code J44.0 (COPD with acute lower respiratory infection) and the pneumonia code is based on the circumstances of the admission.

When **influenza is associated with pneumonia**, an influenza/pneumonia combination code is sequenced first followed by the pneumonia code.

Lobar pneumonia (J18.1) should only be coded when the provider specifically documents "lobar pneumonia" and a causal organism is not specified. See Coding Clinic 2019 Third Quarter, p.37.

For pneumonia due to **vaping**, assign code U07.0, Vaping-related disorder as the principal diagnosis, with additional codes for the pneumonia or other manifestations. For lung injury due to vaping, assign only U07.0.

Assign code J69.0 for **aspiration bronchitis** (rather than J68.0) per Coding Clinic 2019 Second Quarter p. 31.

For *DRG Tips*, see DRGs 193-195, Simple pneumonia, and DRGs 177-179, Respiratory infections.

References

• Management of Adults with Hospital-acquired and Ventilator-associated Pneumonia: 2016 Clinical Practice Guidelines by the ISDA and ATS

• Diagnosis and Treatment of Adults with Community-acquired Pneumonia. An Official Clinical Practice Guideline of the ATS and ISDA

• Community-Acquired Pneumonia Requiring Hospitalization among U.S. Adults. NEJM 2015

• Health Care-Associated Pneumonia (HCAP): A Critical Appraisal to Improve Identification, Management and Outcomes

• UpToDate.com: Clinical evaluation and diagnostic testing for community-acquired pneumonia in adults

• UpToDate.com: Aspiration Pneumonia in Adults

• Medscape: Aspiration Pneumonia and Pneumonitis.

DEFINITION

Abnormal accumulation of air within the pleural space between the lung and chest wall. It may occur spontaneously, due to trauma, or as a complication of a procedure. Most cases are self-sealing leaks that limit the size and severity.

There are different types of pneumothorax depending on the cause:

- Spontaneous: occurs spontaneously without any particular precipitating cause, sometimes recurrently.
- Postprocedural (iatrogenic): An unexpected procedural complication as with thoracentesis or chest surgery.
- Tension: caused by an uncontrolled air leak that continues to accumulate, compressing the lung and severely compromising oxygenation. Potentially life-threatening medical emergency.
- Traumatic: due to or following trauma and not the result of a procedure.
- Hemopneumothorax: accumulation of blood and air in the pleural space typically due to trauma.

DIAGNOSTIC CRITERIA

Symptoms are shortness of breath and pleuritic pain. Severe cases may cause extreme respiratory distress and even cyanosis before proceeding to respiratory arrest.

Typically diagnosed with chest x-ray or point-of-care pleural ultrasound and occasionally chest CT scan showing air between a partially deflated lung and the chest wall. Mediastinal shift and complete lung deflation are seen with tension pneumothorax.

TREATMENT

Ranges from simple observation of respiratory status with serial x-rays to chest tube (thoracostomy tube) depending on severity and circumstances.

CODING AND DOCUMENTATION CHALLENGES

A pneumothorax that occurs postprocedurally or iatrogenic pneumothorax is coded to J95.811. Iatrogenic literally means "caused by a doctor" thereby defining it as a complication.

A small postop pneumothorax lasting a short period of time and not requiring prolonged treatment is intrinsic to VATS and open thoracotomy. It should not be coded unless there is specific mention of puncture or laceration of lung or if documented as iatrogenic or as a complication of the procedure.

Postop air leak (J95.812) and other or persistent air leaks (J93.82) clinically describe circumstances causing what would be a pneumothorax, but usually only occur when the patient already has pneumothorax requiring a thoracostomy tube or a "routine" postop thoracostomy tube is in place.

If an air leak or "persistent" air leak follows a procedure, then it is probably unexpected and likely a complication (J95.812). However, air leaks, whether persistent or not, can occur in other circumstances that are not complications including spontaneous and traumatic pneumothorax, and physician clarification may be necessary.

The pneumothorax codes are CCs; hemopneumothorax (code S27.2XXA) and tension pneumothorax (J93.0) are MCCs.

References

- Management of Persistent Air Leaks. Dugan, KC et al. Chest 2017; 152: 417–423
- www.UpToDate: Clinical presentation and diagnosis of pneumothorax
- Hemothorax: medscape.com

DEFINITION

Pulmonary hypertension is elevated pulmonary artery blood pressure.

Pulmonary heart disease (PHD), or "cor pulmonale," is the consequence of pulmonary hypertension causing right heart failure (initially diastolic but may progress to systolic). PHD is the current preferred terminology instead of cor pulmonale, but cor pulmonale is still widely used.

Acute PHD is usually due to acute pulmonary embolism or acute exacerbation of an underlying cause of chronic pulmonary hypertension and PHD.

Chronic pulmonary hypertension and PHD are either primary (hereditary or idiopathic) or secondary commonly due to COPD, interstitial lung disease including pulmonary fibrosis, obstructive sleep apnea, cystic fibrosis, and severe left heart disease.

Other causes include chronic hypoxic states, chronic pulmonary embolism, other chronic pulmonary disease, medication/drug induced, HIV infection, connective tissue diseases (like SLE, rheumatoid arthritis, scleroderma), sickle cell disease, and sarcoidosis.

DIAGNOSTIC CRITERIA

Pulmonary hypertension: Mean pulmonary artery pressure (MPAP) >20 mmHg.

Pulmonary heart disease is typically characterized by

- Pulmonary hypertension
- An associated underlying condition causing pulmonary hypertension (except primary pulmonary hypertension)
- Physical exam: neck vein distension; peripheral edema; evidence of severe chronic lung disease
- Doppler echocardiogram:
  - *Chronic*: pulmonary hypertension, right ventricular hypertrophy or dilatation, right ventricular diastolic dysfunction, tricuspid insufficiency, pulmonic valve insufficiency.
  - *Acute*: right heart (ventricular) strain or dilatation; increased PA pressure from baseline (if known).

TREATMENT

Includes management of the underlying cause, supplemental oxygen, and cautious use of diuretics (over-diuresis can cause decompensation). Calcium channel blockers and PDE-5 inhibitors, like Cialis and Viagra, are sometimes prescribed for pulmonary hypertension and PHD because they significantly reduce pulmonary artery blood pressure.

CODING AND DOCUMENTATION CHALLENGES

Pulmonary hypertension is not a CC unless specified as primary (group 1) pulmonary hypertension (code I27.0) which is uncommon.

ICD-10 does not recognize that pulmonary heart disease and cor pulmonale are synonymous clinical terms. Pulmonary heart disease, acute, chronic, or unspecified, is assigned to code I27.9, Pulmonary heart disease, unspecified, a non-CC. Chronic cor pulmonale (or unspecified) is assigned to code I27.81, a non-CC.

Although the ICD-10 Index assigns "**acute cor pulmonale**" to code I26.09, Other pulmonary embolism with acute cor pulmonale, Coding Clinic 2014 Fourth Quarter states that because code I26.09 is titled "Other pulmonary embolism with acute cor pulmonale," it is not appropriate to use this combination code since the patient does not have pulmonary embolism.

Unfortunately, ICD-10 has still made no provision for acute pulmonary heart disease or acute cor pulmonale due to other causes. However, the DRG definitions allow code I26.09, when sequenced as principal diagnosis, to serve as its own MCC resulting in DRG 175.

However, patients with acute cor pulmonale do have **acute diastolic right heart failure** (see *Heart Failure*) which could be the best opportunity to capture the severity of illness associated with pulmonary heart disease and acute cor pulmonale when unrelated to pulmonary embolism.

On the other hand, patients with **chronic pulmonary embolism** requiring long-term anticoagulants would be coded to I27.82 (CC). Code I27.82 would be used, rather than Z86.711 (history of pulmonary embolism), when recurrent episodes have occurred that require lifelong anticoagulant therapy. The diagnosis is a subjective clinical one taking into account the number and frequency of episodes. Placement of a Greenfield filter strongly suggests chronic pulmonary embolism. Code Z86.711 would be used when an episode of acute pulmonary embolism has clinically resolved (about 1-2 weeks) even though anticoagulants are continued for 3-12 months to prevent a recurrence.

References

- State of the art summary on diagnosis, prognosis, therapy and future perspectives of pulmonary hypertension. European Respiratory Journal 2019
- The Merck Manual: Cor Pulmonale
- UpToDate.com: Pulmonary hypertension due to lung disease and/or hypoxemia (group 3 hypertension): Epidemiology, pathogenesis, and diagnostic evaluation in adults
- UpToDate.com: Treatment of pulmonary arterial hypertension (group 1) in adults: Pulmonary hypertension-specific therapy
- Medscape: Pulmonary Arterial Hypertension
- Coding Clinic 2017 Fourth Quarter p. 14
- Coding Clinic 2014 Fourth Quarter p. 21.

DEFINITION

Respiratory failure: Significant abnormality in blood gases primarily resulting from inadequate ventilation or impaired alveolar gas (O_2, CO_2) exchange often requiring respiratory support.

Respiratory arrest: Cessation of or agonal respirations necessitating mechanical ventilation.

Neonatal respiratory distress syndrome (NRDS): NRDS is usually due to hyaline membrane disease caused by deficiency of surfactant resulting in collapse of alveoli. Inadequate clearance of lung fluid also plays a role. Almost always associated with respiratory failure.

Meconium aspiration syndrome: Serious life-threatening condition that occurs when an infant inhales a mixture of meconium and amniotic fluid, preventing the infant from receiving adequate oxygen.

Primary sleep apnea: Reduction or pauses in breathing that occur during sleep. Also known as congenital central hypoventilation syndrome.

Other apnea: Apnea from other causes including obstructive apnea unrelated to sleep and "apnea of prematurity." May or may not be associated with respiratory failure.

Transient tachypnea (TTN): A self-limited condition commonly seen in full-term neonates due to excessive fluid accumulation in the lungs.

Cyanotic attack: Neonatal cyanosis, particularly central cyanosis. Usually has an underlying cause but may go unexplained.

DIAGNOSTIC CRITERIA

Respiratory failure: Pediatricians rely heavily on signs, symptoms, imaging and precipitating factors and management requirements for diagnosis. See ***Respiratory Failure—Pediatric*** for further explanation to support the diagnosis.

ABG may not be obtained and oxygen saturation by pulse oximetry (SpO2) is often relied upon. Most neonates with respiratory failure need to be intubated for mechanical ventilation, but it is not an absolute requirement for diagnosis.

Neonatal respiratory distress syndrome: Infant exhibits signs such as tachypnea, grunting, with increased oxygen demand. Chest x-ray is typically abnormal showing hypoaeration of lungs and bilateral fine granular opacities ("ground glass appearance") or air bronchograms. Mild cases treated with oxygen, more severe require intubation and surfactant administration.

Transient tachypnea: Tachypnea in full-term neonates without other findings. Blood oxygenation is usually not impaired. The exact cause is unknown. Must be observed for development of respiratory fatigue or failure.

Cyanotic attack: Cyanosis associated with significant and potentially life-threatening diseases due to cardiac, metabolic, neurologic, infectious, and pulmonary disorders almost always associated with some respiratory distress. Usually has an underlying cause but may go unexplained.

TREATMENT

Directed at underlying causes plus supplemental oxygen and respiratory support like CPAP, BiPAP, SiPAP (Synchronized Intermittent Positive Airway Pressure), or mechanical ventilation as indicated.

CODING AND DOCUMENTATION CHALLENGES

All of the neonate respiratory abnormalities described above and listed below move the MS-DRG from 795 (Normal newborn) to higher-weighted MS-DRGs 794 (Neonates with other significant problems), 793 (Full term neonate with major problems) and 790 (Extreme immaturity or respiratory distress syndrome, neonate).

The following are the newborn respiratory abnormalities with ICD-10 codes:

Diagnosis	Code
Transient tachypnea	P22.1
Respiratory distress, unspecified	P22.9
Meconium aspiration w/o resp symptoms	P24.00
Cyanotic attack	P28.2
Other specified newborn respiratory conditions	P28.89
Primary sleep apnea	P28.3
Other apnea	P28.4
Meconium aspiration w resp symptoms	P24.01
Respiratory distress syndrome	P22.0
Respiratory failure or insufficiency	P28.5
Respiratory arrest	P28.81

The first five codes, when assigned as a secondary diagnosis with Z38--, are assigned to APR-DRG 640 (Normal newborn) but with SOI 2. The other codes are assigned to APR-DRGs for neonates with other significant conditions or major respiratory conditions.

Meconium stained amniotic fluid at birth creates the risk for aspiration and requires careful monitoring for possible meconium aspiration syndrome (P24.01).

Non-invasive ventilation, such as CPAP (5A09357), should not be coded if only briefly administered to a newborn for resuscitation purposes.

References

- Medscape.com: Pediatric Respiratory Failure
- UpToDate.com: Acute respiratory distress in children: Emergency evaluation and initial stabilization
- UpToDate.com: Overview of cyanosis in the newborn
- UpToDate.com: Overview of neonatal respiratory distress: Disorders of transition
- Non-invasive Ventilation in Premature Infants: Based on Evidence or Habit. J Clin Neonatol. 2013; 2: 155–159
- Coding Clinic 2017 First Quarter p. 29.

DEFINITION

Respiratory failure is classified as hypoxemic (low arterial oxygen levels), hypercapnic (elevated levels of carbon dioxide gas), or a combination of the two. In most cases one or the other predominates.

Respiratory failure is classified into two types:

- **Hypoxemic (Type 1): pO2 < 60 mmHg with normal or subnormal pCO2.** *Impaired oxygen* exchange in the alveoli, as in COPD, pneumonia, pulmonary edema, or pulmonary embolism.

- **Hypercapnic (Type 2): pCO2 > 50 mmHg.** *Impaired ventilation,* primarily in COPD, requires increased effort to ventilate the lungs, and characterized by hypercapnia with variable degrees of hypoxemia.

The diagnosis and classification of respiratory failure is based on blood gas measurements: arterial blood gas (ABG) and pulse oximetry (SpO2). See the following **Blood Gas Measurements** which includes venous blood gas measurement.

Respiratory failure is also categorized as acute, chronic and acute-on-chronic depending on its onset, degree of blood gas abnormalities, and duration. For guidance on patients with chronic and acute-on-chronic respiratory failure, see **Respiratory Failure–Chronic** that follows.

SYMPTOMS

Any patient with acute respiratory failure would be expected to exhibit some degree of respiratory difficulty.

This may be nothing more than dyspnea or tachypnea (respirations > 20), wheezing, or decreased respirations (< 10), but may progress to severe symptoms like labored breathing, accessory muscle use, retractions, cyanosis and eventually respiratory arrest. Confusion and somnolence are not uncommon.

DIAGNOSTIC CRITERIA

Acute hypoxemic respiratory failure

- pO2 < 60 mmHg on <u>room air</u> measured by ABG, or
- SpO2 < 91% on <u>room air</u> measured by pulse oximetry, or
- P/F ratio < 300 on oxygen

The above pO2 and SpO2 criteria are based on room air measurements. When room air values are not available or when the degree of respiratory failure needs to be determined after oxygen therapy is initiated, calculate the P/F ratio.

Acute hypercapnic respiratory failure

- pCO2 > 50 mmHg with pH < 7.35

The diagnosis requires an ABG (or venous blood gas) demonstrating an elevated pCO2 due to acute retention/accumulation of carbon dioxide gas resulting in acidic pH < 7.35 (respiratory acidosis).

Note*: pO2 and PaO2 are synonymous, as are pCO2 and PaCO2.*

In some cases like head trauma, drug overdose, or over-sedation, the brain's respiratory center is suppressed causing reduced respiratory drive with decreased ventilation that may progress to **respiratory arrest**. In these cases, hypercapnic respiratory failure usually precedes hypoxemic respiratory failure.

Acute respiratory distress syndrome (ARDS), also known as acute lung injury (ALI), is a life-threatening lung condition caused by severe systemic insults. ARDS is recognized by acute hypoxemic respiratory failure (P/F ratio < 300), characteristic chest x-ray showing bilateral symmetrical pulmonary edema, and an acute inciting event such as severe traumatic injury, sepsis, prolonged shock, aspiration, drug overdose, cardiothoracic surgery, and acute pancreatitis. Typically requires intensive care and mechanical ventilation.

P/F RATIO

The P/F ratio is a powerful objective tool to identify acute hypoxemic respiratory failure when supplemental oxygen is already being administered, and no room air ABG or SpO2 is available. A P/F ratio < 300 confirms hypoxemic respiratory failure because it is equivalent to room air pO2 < 60 mmHg.

The P/F ratio cannot be used in the setting of chronic hypoxemic respiratory failure on home O2 since it is always < 300. Similarly, pO2 and SpO2 are not valid on room air for such patients, but can be applied to them while breathing oxygen at their usual home flow rate or higher. See *Respiratory Failure–Chronic & Acute-on-Chronic*.

P/F RATIO CALCULATION: PAO2 DIVIDED BY FIO2

"P" represents PaO2 (arterial pO2) from the ABG. "F" represents the FIO2 – the fraction (percent) of inspired oxygen that the patient is receiving expressed as a decimal (40% oxygen = FIO2 of 0.40). P divided by F = P/F ratio.

EXAMPLE A patient has a pO2 of 70 mmHg while receiving 36% oxygen (4 liters/min). The P/F ratio = 70 divided by 0.36 = 194 (severe acute respiratory failure).

A P/F ratio of 194 represents a pO2 of 39 mmHg on room air, well below 60 mmHg on room air.

The P/F ratio indicates what the PaO2 would be on room air if oxygen were discontinued.

P/F Ratio	Equivalent to a pO2 on room air of	Condition
≥ 400	≥ 80	Normal
< 400	60-79	Hypoxemia
< 300	50-59	Respiratory failure
< 250	40-49	Severe respiratory failure
< 200	< 40	Critical respiratory failure

P/F ratio using SpO2. When the pO2 is unknown because an ABG was not performed, pulse oximetry readings (SpO2) can be used to calculate the P/F ratio. The SpO2 can be used as a surrogate to approximate the pO2 as shown below:

SpO2 (percent)	pO2 (mm Hg)
86	51
87	52
88	54
89	56
90	58
91	60

SpO2 (percent)	pO2 (mm Hg)
92	64
93	68
94	73
95	80
96	90
97	110

EXAMPLE A patient has an SpO2 of 95% on 4 liters of oxygen. Based on this information, the SpO2 of 95% is equal to a pO2 of 80 mmHg. Four liters/min of oxygen represents an FIO2 = 0.36. P/F ratio = 80 / 0.36 = 222.

Although the patient may be stable and asymptomatic receiving 36% oxygen, the patient still has acute respiratory failure. If supplemental oxygen were withdrawn, the room air pO2 would only be 40 mmHg, significantly less than the diagnostic criteria of < 60 mmHg on room air.

O2 flow rate to FIO2. A nasal cannula provides oxygen at adjustable flow rates in liters of oxygen per minute (L/min or LPM). The actual FIO2 (percent oxygen) delivered by nasal cannula is somewhat variable and less reliable than with a mask but can be estimated by increasing 4% for each L/min flow. Assume room air is 20% (0.20), 1 L=0.24, 2L=0.28, 3L=0.32, 4L=0.36, 5L=0.40.

Sepsis. The P/F ratio is one of the SOFA score diagnostic criteria for Sepsis-3. A P/F ratio of 300-399 indicates hypoxemia and equals one point on the SOFA scale; < 300 represents hypoxemic respiratory failure equaling two points if baseline is above 400. For Sepsis-2, the acute respiratory failure criterion for severe sepsis is a P/F <300.

BLOOD GAS MEASUREMENTS

Arterial blood gas (ABG) and pulse oximetry (SpO2) are two methods of measuring blood gases. These are defined as:

Measure	Definition	Normal
pO2	Partial pressure of oxygen, or oxygen content, in mmHg	≥ 80
pCO2	Partial pressure of carbon dioxide, or carbon dioxide content, in mmHg	35 – 45
pH	Measure of the degree of acidity	7.35 – 7.45
SaO2	Oxygen saturation (percent of hemoglobin carrying oxygen) as reported on ABG and is relatively proportional with pO2	≥ 95%
SpO2	Oxygen saturation (percent of hemoglobin carrying oxygen) as measured by pulse oximetry and is relatively proportional with pO2	≥ 95%
FIO2	Percent of supplemental oxygen expressed as a decimal, e.g., 40% oxygen = 0.40.	Room air 20% = 0.20
P/F ratio	pO2 / FIO2	≥ 400

Degrees of Hypoxemia

Measure	Normal	Hypoxemia	Respiratory failure
pO2 (room air)	≥ 80 mmHg	60-79 mmHg	< 60 mmHg
SpO2 (room air)	≥ 95%	91-94%	< 91%
P/F Ratio (on oxygen)	≥ 400	300-399	< 300

Venous Blood Gas (VBG). The venous blood gas is an alternative method of *estimating* systemic pCO2 and pH that avoids the need for arterial puncture. VBG can be used for the diagnosis and management of hypercapnic respiratory failure or acid-base disorders. The venous pH is usually 0.02-0.05 pH units lower than arterial pH and venous pCO2 about 3-8 mmHg higher than arterial PCO2.

Taking these adjustments into account, providers may apply the usual acute hypercapnic respiratory failure criteria: arterial $pCO_2 > 50 +$ pH < 7.35.

The venous pO_2 cannot be used for the diagnosis of hypoxemic respiratory failure or other clinical purposes because it is highly variable and much lower than arterial pO_2. However, SpO_2 can be used to identify hypoxemic respiratory failure combined with VBG for the hypercapnic component.

TREATMENT AND MANAGEMENT

Patients with acute respiratory failure are always treated and managed with supplemental oxygen together with other measures to correct hypoventilation including steroids (Solumedrol), inhaled bronchodilators, mucolytics and respiratory therapy.

The diagnosis of respiratory failure is based on blood gases and not on how much oxygen is required to maintain adequate oxygenation. Some hospitalized patients require no more than 28% oxygen; others may require up to 100%.

Supplemental oxygen may be administered by mask or nasal cannula. A nasal cannula provides oxygen at adjustable flow rates in liters of oxygen per minute (L/min or LPM). The actual FIO_2 (percent oxygen) delivered by nasal cannula is somewhat variable and less reliable than with a mask but can be estimated as shown below increasing 4% for each liter/min flow. Room air is assumed to be FIO_2 of 20%, or 0.20.

Flow Rate (liter/min)	FIO2
1	0.24
2	0.28
3	0.32
4	0.36
5	0.40
6	0.44

A Venturi (Venti-mask) mask delivers oxygen at predictable and reliable FIO2 values ranging from 0.24 to 0.50. A nonrebreather (NRB) mask is designed to deliver approximately 100% oxygen.

A patient who requires 36% oxygen or more, mechanical ventilation, or initiation of BiPAP nearly always has acute respiratory failure, but these measures are not required to establish the diagnosis.

Intubation for airway protection. Patients with a severely altered level of consciousness may have lost their "gag" reflex that helps protect the airway from aspiration of regurgitated stomach contents or upper airway accumulation of blood or secretions and are intubated and ventilated for "airway protection." Familiar clinical situations are head trauma, CVA, brain hemorrhage and drug overdose.

Some of these patients may be able to maintain pulmonary ventilation and acceptable blood gases without ventilation support, but require intubation and mechanical ventilation for "airway protection" only. Others may also have suppression of the brain stem respiratory center resulting in hypoventilation and causing accumulation of carbon dioxide (hypercapnic respiratory failure) and eventually hypoxemia as well.

Deciding when respiratory failure should be queried or is a clinically valid diagnosis in this situation can be challenging. To validate respiratory failure:

- Check pre-intubation blood gases as usual for acute respiratory failure
- Check post-intubation P/F ratio. If < 300 = acute respiratory failure
- Documentation of apnea or extremely low respiratory rate < 10 ("ventilatory failure")

Without such substantiating evidence, the diagnosis may be challenged as clinically invalid. The fact that the patient would develop respiratory failure if not intubated does not necessarily qualify it for code assignment if it never actually occurred.

On the other hand, it may be that after intubation such a patient subsequently develops genuine hypoxemic respiratory failure substantiated by a P/F ratio < 300. In this case, documentation or query is appropriate since the diagnosis would be clinically valid at that point.

CODING AND DOCUMENTATION CHALLENGES

Physicians often have the false impression that because the patient's symptoms are relieved and the pO2 and/or SpO2 have improved with supplemental oxygen, respiratory failure has resolved.

Even though symptoms are relieved and oxygenation improved or normalized with oxygen administration, the underlying respiratory failure persists which would become obvious if oxygen were removed. A P/F ratio < 300 confirms continuing respiratory failure without having to discontinue oxygen. Serial P/F ratios can also monitor progression during oxygen administration and may detect early deterioration.

An exacerbation of symptoms requiring an increase in chronic supplemental oxygen indicates an "acute exacerbation" of chronic respiratory failure and classified as acute-on-chronic respiratory failure if properly documented. See *Respiratory Failure–Chronic & Acute-on-Chronic* that follows.

Respiratory failure unspecified (J96.90) is an MCC just like acute, and specification of acute, hypoxemic or hypercapnic is unnecessary. Before assigning code J96.90, be sure the diagnostic criteria for acute respiratory failure are met to distinguish from chronic respiratory failure.

Respiratory insufficiency (code R06.89, a symptom code) is a non-specific, undefined term that is probably intended to describe hypoxemia (pO2 60-79 or SpO2 91-94%) without respiratory failure. Query for respiratory failure if criteria are met. If postoperative, see also *Respiratory Failure–Postprocedural*.

Hypercapnic respiratory failure may be improperly diagnosed as "**respiratory acidosis**" (acid-base disorder) which always accompanies it and represents the same blood gas abnormality. However, the code for "respiratory acidosis" (E87.2) is a CC in contrast to the MCC status of hypercapnic respiratory failure, hence the need for clarification.

Code J80 (MCC) is used for ARDS. Since ARDS is always associated with hypoxemic respiratory failure, respiratory failure is not separately coded. Do not confuse acute respiratory distress (R0603) with ARDS.

The P/F ratio should be included on ABG reports to assist clinicians and to further support the diagnosis of respiratory failure, but often is not. Typically a software change using the simple P/F formula is necessary. It is also important to educate the nursing staff to always include the L/min of oxygen with all SpO2 recordings.

Coding Clinics 1988 Third Quarter p. 7 and 1990 Second Quarter p. 20 support the definition and the diagnostic criteria for hypoxemic and hypercapnic respiratory failure discussed above but do not mention the P/F ratio.

References

• Respiratory Failure: NCBI Bookshelf. National Library of Medicine, National Institutes of Health, August 2020

• Management of Acute Ventilatory Failure. Postgrad Med J 2006; 82: 438–445

• Medscape: Respiratory Failure

• The American-European Consensus Conference on ARDS. Am J Respir Crit Care Med 1994; 149: 818–824

• An equation for the oxygen hemoglobin dissociation curve. J Appl Physiol 1973; 35: 570–571

• Surviving Sepsis Campaign: International Guidelines for Management of Severe Sepsis and Septic Shock: 2017

• Acute respiratory distress syndrome: the Berlin Definition. JAMA 2012;307:2526-33

• UpToDate.com: The evaluation, diagnosis and treatment of the adult patient with acute hypercapnic respiratory failure

• UpToDate.com: Venous blood gases and other alternatives to arterial blood gas.

DEFINITION

Chronic respiratory failure is caused by abnormalities of oxygenation and carbon dioxide elimination due to chronic lung disease. It may be classified as hypoxemic or hypercapnic.

Common causes include severe COPD, pulmonary fibrosis, interstitial lung disease, cystic fibrosis and end-stage heart failure.

DIAGNOSTIC CRITERIA

- Hypoxemic: SpO2 < 91% on room air (or pO2 < 60), and/or
- Hypercapnic: Chronic hypercapnea (elevated pCO2 > 50) with normal pH (7.35 – 7.45)

The use of home oxygen is a reliable indicator of chronic hypoxemic respiratory failure since SpO2 ≤ 88% is required to meet medical necessity criteria.

TREATMENT

Home O2 for chronic hypoxemic respiratory failure. Optimal management of underlying cause for both types.

ACUTE-ON-CHRONIC RESPIRATORY FAILURE

Most patients who are admitted with respiratory distress in the setting of chronic respiratory failure would be expected to have acute-on-chronic respiratory failure.

Acute-on-chronic hypoxemic respiratory failure is an acute exacerbation or decompensation of chronic respiratory failure recognized by worsening dyspnea and the following:

- Increase in chronic supplemental oxygen, or
- Decrease in baseline pO2 by > 10mmHg on ABG, or
- pO2 < 60 or SpO2 < 91% on usual home O2 (rather than room air)

> **EXAMPLE** Patient on home O2 at 2L/min admitted with dyspnea and SpO2 of 93% on 4L/min. The SpO2 on usual home O2 (2L/min) is expected to be > 91%.
>
> This patient now requires 4L/min to maintain SpO2 at 93% (just barely above 91%) indicating acute exacerbation of chronic hypoxemic respiratory failure. Pt discharged with a SpO2 of 92% on 2 liters provides further confirmation.

Acute-on-chronic hypercapnic respiratory failure is recognized by worsening dyspnea and either of the following:

- pCO2 > 50 mmHg with pH < 7.35, or

- Increase in baseline pCO2 on ABG by ≥ 10 mmHg (although baseline pCO2 is rarely available)

CODING AND DOCUMENTATION CHALLENGES

While the use of home oxygen is a reliable indicator of chronic hypoxemic respiratory failure, it can be difficult to identify chronic hypercapnic respiratory failure without an ABG to confirm.

It is important to note that **most patients with COPD** *do not have chronic respiratory failure* since their baseline SpO2 is > 91% and/or home oxygen is not required. They do not always have "chronically lower PaO2 [or SpO2] and an increased PaCO2" as mentioned in a 1988 Coding Clinic that audit contractors frequently cite.

When COPD patients who do not require home oxygen and therefore do not have chronic hypoxemic respiratory failure are admitted with a PaO2 < 60 or SpO2 < 91%, they do meet the diagnostic criteria for acute respiratory failure. In addition, the room air SpO2 is expected to return to baseline (> 91%) by discharge without any need for home oxygen.

> **EXAMPLES** Patient with COPD not on home O2 admitted with dyspnea and ABG pH 7.46, PO2 65, PCO2 36 (low normal) on 3 liters O2. On discharge her SpO2 = 95% on room air. P/F ratio = 203 (65/0.32) which meets the criteria for acute respiratory failure. The admission PCO2 of 36 proves there is no chronic hypercapnic respiratory failure as well.

On the other hand, consider a patient who is not on home O2 admitted with an acute exacerbation of COPD and ABG showing a pO2 of 65 on 3 liters, and subsequently discharged essentially unchanged with a SpO2 of 93% on 3 liters home oxygen (equivalent to a pO2 of 68 mmHg). This patient did not have acute respiratory failure but rather most likely had unrecognized chronic hypoxemic respiratory failure.

For patients with chronic respiratory failure on home oxygen, the SpO2 at discharge on their usual home oxygen can help to confirm a pO2 decrease of > 10 mmHg. To illustrate:

EXAMPLE   Patient with chronic respiratory failure on 3 L home O2 is admitted with respiratory distress and an ABG PO2 of 54 on 3 liters. Three days prior to admission the patient was discharged from the ED with an SpO2 of 96% on 3 liters. The patient was treated with 4-5 liters of oxygen during the hospitalization.

Since home O2 is adjusted to keep the SpO2 > 91% (= pO2 > 60), 54 clearly represents an acute decompensation.

When pO2 is unavailable, SpO2 can be used to approximate both the baseline and current pO2. In this example:

- ED discharge baseline: SpO2 96% = pO2 of 90 on 3 liters
- On admission: pO2 of 54 on 3 liters
- Difference: 36 (90 minus 54) on the same O2 flow rate - much more than 10 mmHg decrease.

Reference
- Acute Exacerbations and Respiratory Failure in Chronic Obstructive Pulmonary Disease. Proc Am Thorac Soc 2008; 5: 530–535.

DEFINITION

Respiratory failure is classified as hypoxemic (low arterial oxygen levels), hypercapnic (elevated levels of carbon dioxide gas), or a combination of both.

Causes include severe asthma, pneumonia, infection, neuromuscular disorders (e.g., Guillain-Barré, spinal cord injury), muscular dystrophy, trauma and others.

DIAGNOSTIC CRITERIA

Signs and symptoms: Pediatricians rely heavily on clinical signs, symptoms, imaging and management requirements to diagnose pediatric respiratory failure, which may be somewhat different from adults.

Common respiratory findings include: Shortness of breath (dyspnea), rapid breathing (tachypnea) for age, decreased respiratory rate ("bradypnea") for age, accessory muscle use, nasal flaring or grunting, head bobbing, belly breathing, retractions or paradoxical chest wall movement (inward with inspiration rather than expansion outward), wheezing and/or stridor, decreased breath sounds, lethargy or inability to feed, cyanosis.

Cardiovascular findings: Tachycardia, bradycardia, hypertension.

Imaging findings: Diffuse interstitial changes, pulmonary edema, extensive lung consolidation; bilateral hyperinflation (severe asthma); large pleural effusions and others.

Age	Tachycardia	Tachypnea	Bradycardia
29 days – 1 year	> 160	> 40	< 100-120
1 – 2 years	> 145	> 40	< 100
2+ – 6 years	> 128	> 30	< 80-90
6+ – 11 years	> 115	> 25	< 65-75
12 –18 years	> 100	> 20	< 60

Hypoxemic respiratory failure. As with adults, the "gold standard" is an ABG showing:

- pO2 < 60 mmHg on room air, or
- P/F ratio < 300 on supplemental oxygen, or
- 10-15 mmHg decrease in pO2 from baseline (if known)

ABGs are not commonly obtained in pediatric patients, and providers rely more on oxygen saturation measured by pulse oximetry (SpO2) for diagnosis and management of hypoxemia. Saturations less than 94% are abnormal but saturations less than 90% are potentially indicative of respiratory failure.

For interpretation of blood gases, P/F ratio and more detailed descriptions of interpreting and applying the above diagnostic criteria, see *Respiratory Failure* for adults.

Hypercapnic respiratory failure. Recognized by elevated pCO2 due to acute retention/accumulation of carbon dioxide gas resulting in an acidic pH < 7.35.

Blood Gases:

- ABG: pCO2 > 50 mmHg with pH < 7.35, or
- Venous blood gases (VBG) or Capillary Blood Gas (CBG) in lieu of ABG
- Capnography: End-tidal CO2 level (ETCO2) > 45 mmHg
- If baseline pCO2 is known, a 10-15 mmHg increase above baseline pCO2

VBG is an alternative method of estimating systemic pCO2 and pH that avoids the need for arterial puncture. VBG can be used for the diagnosis and management of hypercapnic respiratory failure or other acid-base disorders. The venous pH is usually 0.02-0.05 pH units lower than arterial pH and venous pCO2 about 3-8 mmHg higher than arterial pCO2.

Taking these adjustments into account, providers may apply the usual hypercapnic respiratory failure criteria: arterial $pCO_2 > 50$ + arterial $pH < 7.35$.

The venous pO_2 cannot be used to assess oxygenation status in hypoxemic respiratory failure or other clinical purposes.

The CBG pO_2 is more accurate than with VBG but does not match ABG. The pO_2 from CBG should be confirmed with the SpO_2.

Capnography measures the CO_2 content of the last air exhaled from the lungs which is essentially equal to alveolar/capillary CO_2. Elevated $ETCO_2$ indicates CO_2 retention characteristic of hypercapnic respiratory failure.

Capnography suffers from some limitations since it is affected by respiratory rate and acid/base disturbance (acidosis or alkalosis). It is used for intubated and non-intubated patients.

Pediatric acute respiratory distress syndrome (PARDS). ARDS, also known as acute lung injury (ALI), is a specific pathologic condition having certain clinical characteristics causing acute respiratory failure. ARDS is due to inflammation and damage to the alveolar membranes causing fluid to leak into the alveolar air spaces that causes hypoxemia.

ARDS diagnostic criteria and management differ between adults and children. Diagnostic standards have not been fully developed, but the best authoritative source is the 2015 Pediatric Acute Respiratory Distress Syndrome: Consensus Conference.

TREATMENT AND MANAGEMENT

- Intubation, BiPAP or CPAP
- High flow oxygen > 30% or > 3L/min
- Intensive, frequent, repeated inhaled respiratory modalities
- Heliox (mixture of helium and oxygen)
- Inhaled nitric oxide

CODING AND DOCUMENTATION CHALLENGES

The diagnosis of acute respiratory failure is not limited to patients who require intubation and mechanical ventilation and/or have an ABG performed.

Physicians may simply identify hypercapnic respiratory failure as "respiratory acidosis," which is the same thing. Unfortunately, "respiratory acidosis" is a CC / SOI-2, in contrast to the MCC / SOI-4 status of respiratory failure—hence the need for clarification.

References

- www.Medscape.com: Pediatric Respiratory Failure: Practice Essentials, Background, Pathophysiology
- ACDIS White Paper: Pediatric Respiratory Failure The Need for Specific Definitions (Oct. 2016)
- Pediatric Acute Respiratory Distress Syndrome: Consensus Recommendations From the Pediatric Acute Lung Injury Consensus Conference. Pediatr Crit Care Med. 2015 June ; 16(5): 428–439

The diagnosis of respiratory failure following surgery has reimbursement and quality of care implications. Postprocedural respiratory failure is a reportable surgical complication and can adversely affect quality scores for both hospital and surgeon.

On the other hand, the diagnosis and coding of postprocedural respiratory failure often results in a significant payment increase to hospitals since it is an MCC. If diagnosed without firm clinical grounds, it may become the basis for improper DRG payment.

The ICD-10 codes for these conditions are located in Intraoperative and Postprocedural Complications and Disorders of Respiratory System, NEC (J95) and are all MCCs:

- J95.1 Acute pulmonary insufficiency following thoracic surgery
- J95.2 Acute pulmonary insufficiency following nonthoracic surgery
- J95.3 Chronic pulmonary insufficiency following surgery
- J95.821 Acute postprocedural respiratory failure
- J95.822 Acute-on-chronic postprocedural respiratory failure

Respiratory failure following surgery due to other underlying conditions. The Tabular listing for J95.82- (acute postprocedural respiratory failure) has an Excludes1 note: "Respiratory failure in other conditions (J96-)." This indicates that codes J95.82- should not be assigned when post-procedural respiratory failure is attributed by the provider to a preexisting or other underlying condition (e.g., severe COPD, heart failure, aspiration pneumonia, pneumothorax).

A similar Excludes1 note at category J96 (Respiratory failure, NEC) includes "Postprocedural respiratory failure (J95.82-)" creating a circular exclusion for which there is no current explanation or coding advice.

Absent any further clarification, it appears that patients who have other preexisting or underlying conditions documented as the cause of respiratory failure following a procedure rather than a direct result of the procedure, may be assigned a code from category J96 (Respiratory failure, NEC) together with the associated condition instead of codes J95.821 and J95.822 for post-procedural respiratory failure.

Only postprocedural respiratory failure codes J95.821 and J95.822 (acute and acute-on-chronic postprocedural respiratory failure) are included in the **PSI-11 Postoperative Respiratory Failure** measure for the CMS pay for performance programs, and are excluded if POA or non-elective surgery (see PSI-11 technical specifications for all exclusions). Codes from category J96 are not included, e.g., J96.00 (acute respiratory failure) and J96.20 (acute on chronic respiratory failure).

Postprocedural respiratory failure not clinically supported. Some physicians have been inclined to document a diagnosis of "respiratory failure" or "pulmonary insufficiency" when patients require ventilator support which is an expected or a routine practice following the procedure with no apparent evidence of an acute pulmonary problem. Such practices may be problematic because the assignment of codes may be an adverse quality indicator and result in improper reimbursement.

To validate the diagnosis, the patient must have acute pulmonary dysfunction requiring non-routine aggressive measures. A patient who requires a short period of routine ventilator support during surgical recovery does not have acute respiratory failure, and a code for it should not be assigned on the claim. To avoid improper code assignment and claim submission, providers should be encouraged not to use such terms in the postoperative setting unless the patient has a significant unexpected respiratory problem.

Pulmonary insufficiency. The diagnosis of pulmonary insufficiency (whether acute, chronic or unspecified) is undefined with no clinical diagnostic standards, which is in contrast to respiratory failure that has clear diagnostic standards. It is certainly not a valid diagnosis for routine post-op management when no significant underlying pulmonary problem can be substantiated; therefore, these codes should be used with caution since coding without a clear definition could expose the hospital to regulatory scrutiny.

DEFINITION

Muscle necrosis with release of creatine kinase (CK) and myoglobin.

Causes include prolonged pressure on muscle tissue interfering with blood flow (e.g., lying immobile after a fall); severe soft tissue/muscle trauma; extreme muscular exertion; adverse effects of medication, alcohol, illicit drugs; certain types of myopathy; viral infections including HIV; sepsis. When severe, it commonly causes AKI due to ATN.

DIAGNOSTIC CRITERIA

- CK levels at presentation are usually 5 times the upper limit of normal, but range from 1,500 to over 100k units/L
  - *Normal reference range is approximately 22 to 198 (up to 300) units/L but depends on gender and lab test used*
- Often with elevated myoglobin in urine and/or serum (reference range 0-85 ng/ml). May not always be detected because it is quickly eliminated.
- Muscle pain occurs in about 50% of cases

TREATMENT

Aggressive IV fluids to prevent ATN. Correction of underlying cause. Correction of any associated electrolyte imbalance (e.g. hyperkalemia, hypo- or hyper-calcemia).

CODING AND DOCUMENTATION CHALLENGES

Urine dipstick may show a "false positive" for blood with no or just a few RBCs (< 5/hpf) reported because both hemoglobin and myoglobin test positive.

AKI in rhabdomyolysis is always due to ATN, although AKI is often documented. For patients admitted with a diagnosis of AKI or ATN due to rhabdomyolysis, AKI/ATN would most likely be the principal diagnosis particularly if it was the focus of treatment.

Rhabdomyolysis is assigned code M62.82 (CC).

Traumatic rhabdomyolysis is coded T79.6XXA (non-CC) and should be reserved for severe soft tissue/muscle injury, not just lying immobile after a fall without significant trauma.

Traumatic rhabdomyolysis is only coded when the provider explicitly documents it as traumatic. Provider clarification may be needed.

References

- UpToDate.com. Clinical features and diagnosis of heme pigment-induced acute kidney injury
- UpToDate.com. Clinical manifestations and diagnosis of rhabdomyolysis
- Coding Clinic 2002 Third Quarter p. 28
- Coding Clinic 2019 Second Quarter p. 12.

DEFINITION

- **Sepsis**: SIRS due to an infection (either suspected or confirmed). Excludes SIRS due to other causes.
- **SIRS**: Systemic inflammatory response syndrome (SIRS) is the body's systemic response to infection or non-infectious causes such as trauma, burns, pancreatitis, major surgery, or other insult/injury.
- **Non-infectious SIRS**: SIRS due to causes other than infection.

DIAGNOSTIC CRITERIA

Infection (either suspected or confirmed), and **some** of the following **not easily explained** by another co-existing condition (other than the infection):

General variables	Hemodynamic variables
• Temp > 38.3C (≥ 101F) or < 36C (<96.8F)	• SBP < 90 or MAP < 70 or SBP decrease > 40
• Heart rate > 90/min	**Organ dysfunction variables**
• Tachypnea (RR > 20)	• P/F ratio < 300
• Altered mental status	• Creatinine increase > 0.5
• Significant edema or positive fluid balance	• Acute oliguria
• Hyperglycemia > 140 in the absence of diabetes	• Ileus (absent bowel sounds)
	• INR > 1.5, or PTT > 60 secs, or thrombocytopenia <100K
Inflammatory variables	• Hyperbilirubinemia > 4
• Leukocytosis: WBC > 12K or < 4K or Bands > 10%	**Tissue perfusion variables**
• C-reactive protein elevated	• Lactate > 1*
• Procalcitonin elevated	• Decreased capillary refill or mottling

Most medical literature does not support Lactate > 1.0 as a sepsis criterion, particularly since a lactate level of 1.0 is in the normal reference range with 1.8-2.0 at the upper limit. The widely held consensus opinion is that > 2.0 should be the indicator for sepsis and > 4.0, equivalent to shock, for severe sepsis.

The use of "**some**" in the definition is usually taken to mean "two or more" but is intended to allow the provider to determine the number applicable to each individual patient based on the clinical circumstances.

The temperature, WBC, lactate level, and persistent hypotension criteria very strongly support the diagnosis of sepsis. Because **tachypnea and tachycardia** are so common in hospitalized patients for many reasons, they should not ordinarily be used as the only two criteria for diagnosing sepsis.

The diagnosis of sepsis depends entirely on the physician's clinical interpretation of these criteria and their significance.

Severe Sepsis:

- **Sepsis** with **associated acute organ dysfunction (**see Organ dysfunction variables)

- **Septic shock**:
  - Refractory hypotension* (SBP < 90, or MAP < 70, or reduction in SBP of > 40) and often requiring vasopressor therapy like dopamine; or
  - Lactate > 4.0

Refractory means persistent hypotension despite effective fluid resuscitation over 1 hour with at least 30 cc/kg of crystalloid (usually normal saline).

TREATMENT

May include IV antibiotics (often broad-spectrum, multiple), aggressive IV fluids to prevent organ failure, supplemental oxygen, careful monitoring of vital signs and organ function, and often intensive care.

CODING AND DOCUMENTATION CHALLENGES

When a patient is admitted with both sepsis and a localized infection, such as pneumonia or cellulitis, sepsis is sequenced first and the code for the localized infection is assigned as a secondary diagnosis (OCG I.C.1.4).

Circumstances in which sepsis is **not** the principal diagnosis include:

- Sepsis or signs/symptoms of sepsis not present on admission.

- Postprocedural sepsis or sepsis due to a device or implant is coded to the appropriate complication code and sequenced first (e.g., T81.44XA, T85.79XA), with additional code(s) to identify any systemic and/or localized infection as a secondary diagnosis.

- Sepsis (even though present on admission) was not the principal reason for admission (did not meet the definition of principal diagnosis).

The publicly reported CMS Inpatient Quality Reporting **SEP-1 severe sepsis core measure** to guide treatment with a standardized order set to lower morbidity and mortality defines severe sepsis as SIRS + acute organ dysfunction using a modified version of the SIRS definition.

Most Medicare Advantage and commercial payors and their auditors have adopted the Sepsis-3 guidelines which requires organ dysfunction or "severe sepsis" as the basis of the diagnosis. Even with documentation of organ dysfunction, many payer auditors are denying the diagnosis of sepsis if the organ dysfunction is not associated with the sepsis by the provider, stating that the organ dysfunction is due to the local infection alone. The severe sepsis code (R65.20) can only be assigned if "severe" sepsis is documented or the organ dysfunction is clearly linked with sepsis.

CDI and coding should consider querying providers to **link / associate the acute organ dysfunction with sepsis** to allow the severe sepsis codes (R65.20, R65.21) to be assigned. For example, "Acute respiratory failure due to sepsis," "Sepsis-related hyperbilirubinemia," or "Hypotension due to sepsis." See also *Sepsis-3.*

Neither the Sepsis-2 or Sepsis-3 Definitions Conferences exclude the P/F ratio criteria for respiratory system organ dysfunction in cases of pneumonia.

SIRS due to an infection ("infectious SIRS") is not indexed and does not have an ICD-10 code. It must be clarified as sepsis. For example, a diagnosis of "SIRS due to pneumonia" can only be coded as "pneumonia" unless sepsis is mentioned in the record.

Bacteremia, code R78.81, means simply a "positive blood culture." Bacteremia cannot be assigned together with sepsis (see Excludes1 note at category A41).

Sepsis and septic shock complicating abortion, pregnancy, childbirth, the puerperium and newborn sepsis are dealt with in OCG sections I.C.15 and I.C.16.f.

References

• 2001 International Sepsis Definitions Conference. Crit Care Med 2003; 31:1250 –1256

• Surviving Sepsis Campaign: International Guidelines for Management of Severe Sepsis and Septic Shock: 2008 and 2012

• 2015 Surviving Sepsis Campaign Updated Bundles in Response to New Evidence

• ICD-10-CM Official Coding Guidelines Sections I.A.15 and I.C.1.d

• Coding Clinic 2014 Third Quarter p. 4

• Coding Clinic 2017 Fourth Quarter p. 98-99.

DEFINITION

Sepsis: Life-threatening organ dysfunction caused by a dysregulated host response to infection (confirmed or suspected).

Septic shock: Persisting hypotension requiring vasopressors to maintain MAP (mean arterial pressure) > 65 mmHg **and** having a serum lactate level > 2 mmol/L despite adequate volume resuscitation.

Sepsis-3 applies only to adults.

DIAGNOSTIC CRITERIA

Organ dysfunction is determined by a two-point increase from baseline of the Sequential (Sepsis-related) Organ Failure Assessment (SOFA) score using six defined organ systems:

1. Respiratory (P/F ratio < 400)*
2. Coagulation (Platelets < 150k)
3. Hepatic (Bilirubin > 1.2)
4. Cardiovascular (MAP < 70)
5. Neurologic (GCS < 15)
6. Renal (Creatinine > 1.2)

Note: The Sepsis-3 definition does not exclude the P/F ratio criteria in cases of pneumonia.

SOFA grades organ dysfunction on a scale of 0 to 4 depending on severity (0 = no dysfunction). The baseline SOFA score for any organ system is assumed to be 0 if the baseline is unknown and the patient has no known preexisting dysfunction in that organ system. Vasopressors include dopamine (DPA), dobutamine, epinephrine, or norepinephrine. See the **SOFA Score Table** that follows.

In simple terms, Sepsis-3 defines sepsis as an uncontrolled systemic inflammatory response due to infection causing acute organ dysfunction — basically the same thing as Sepsis-2 severe sepsis. Organ dysfunction is determined by using the SOFA table.

Sepsis-3 includes a bedside prompt, **qSOFA (quickSOFA)**, to identify patients with infection who are at greater risk for poor outcomes outside the ICU. It is NOT a diagnostic standard for sepsis, and if positive the full SOFA score should be obtained. It is defined as the presence of two or more of three clinical criteria: (1) altered mentation (GCS < 15), (2) respiratory rate ≥ 22, and (3) systolic blood pressure ≤ 100 mm Hg.

In a special article published in October 2021, the Surviving Sepsis Campaign strongly recommends against using qSOFA as a screening tool for sepsis compared with SIRS criteria, which have been shown to be a more accurate predictor of likely sepsis.

CODING AND DOCUMENTATION CHALLENGES

The Sepsis-3 definition was published in the Journal of the American Medical Association (JAMA) in February 2016, defining sepsis as "life-threatening organ dysfunction" due to infection (confirmed or suspected) and discarding the concept of sepsis as SIRS due to infection. In March 2017, the Surviving Sepsis Campaign (SSC) officially adopted the Sepsis-3 definition and criteria as the clinically authoritative diagnostic standard for sepsis.

Nevertheless, widespread skepticism and criticism still exist in the general medical community about changing the diagnostic standard from Sepsis-2 to Sepsis-3. Many providers may disagree professionally with the Sepsis-3 standard and continue to use Sepsis-2 criteria.

Sepsis-3 has been endorsed by the Society of Critical Care Medicine and American Thoracic Society, but not endorsed by the American College of Emergency Physicians, Society of Academic Emergency Medicine, American College of Chest Physicians, or Infectious Disease Society of America due to serious scientific and clinical concerns. All of these medical organizations had originally endorsed Sepsis-2.

Whatever the case may be, most commercial payers and Medicare Advantage plans and their auditors have adopted the Sepsis-3 guidelines.

Medical staff engagement and education is essential to implement Sepsis-3 diagnostic standards. Operationalizing Sepsis-3 can be challenging. While some EHRs calculate the SOFA score, it does not provide the baseline SOFA score and could be misleading since it's the change that matters. Someone would have to be responsible for confirming the score based on the "baseline" clinical information for comparison. For example, a patient with preexisting CKD and baseline creatinine of 1.5 could not be counted as a point towards the SOFA score unless elevated to 2.0 or more.

To ensure early, accurate diagnosis with full SOFA scoring, the total bilirubin, Glasgow Coma Scale (GCS) and P/F ratio should be captured for all patients with an infection. The P/F ratio should be included on ABG reports to assist clinicians and also supports the diagnosis of respiratory failure.

The Sepsis-3 criteria have not changed ICD-10 or OCG guidance. A sepsis code may be assigned if sepsis is documented. Although Sepsis-3 requires organ dysfunction as the basis of the diagnosis, a severe sepsis code (R65.20) can only be assigned if "severe" sepsis is documented or the **organ dysfunction is clearly linked with sepsis**. Many payer auditors are denying the diagnosis of sepsis if the organ dysfunction is not associated with the sepsis by the provider, stating that the organ dysfunction is due to the local infection alone.

CDI and coding should consider querying providers to **link / associate** the acute organ dysfunction with sepsis to allow the severe sepsis codes (R65.20, R65.21) to be assigned. For example, "Acute respiratory failure due to sepsis," "Sepsis-related hyperbilirubinemia," or "Hypotension due to sepsis."

For *DRG Tips*, see DRGs 871-872, Septicemia or severe sepsis.

References
- Singer, M et al; The Third International Consensus Definitions for Sepsis and Septic Shock (Sepsis-3). JAMA 2016; 315: 801-810.

- Rhodes, A. Surviving Sepsis Campaign: International Guidelines for Management of Sepsis and Septic Shock: 2016. Crit Care Med 2017; 45: 486-552
- Prognostic Accuracy of the Quick Sequential Organ Failure Assessment for Mortality in Patients With Suspected Infection: A Systematic Review and Meta-analysis. Ann Intern Med 2018; 168: 266-275
- CMS SEP-1 IQR Measure: Severe Sepsis and Septic Shock Management Bundle 2017
- Coding Clinic 2017 Fourth Quarter p. 98: Severe Sepsis and Acute Organ Dysfunction/Failure

Sepsis-3 SOFA Scale
Acute change due to infection: Score ≥ 2 points

OBJECTIVE MEASUREMENT	POINTS				
	0	1	2	3	4
Respiratory PAO2/FIO2	≥ 400	< 400	< 300	< 200 with resp support	< 100 with resp support
Coagulation Platelet count	≥ 150,000	< 150,000	< 100,000	< 50,000	< 20,000
Hepatic Bilirubin (mg/dL)	< 1.2	1.2-1.9	2.0-5.9	6.0-11.9	> 12.0
Cardiovascular MAP (mmHg) or vasopressor	MAP ≥ 70	MAP < 70	DPA ≤ 5	DPA 5.1-15	DPA >15
Neurologic Glasgow Coma Scale Score	15	13-14	10-12	6-9	< 6
Renal Creatinine (mg/dL) or urine output	< 1.2 -	1.2-1.9 -	2.0-3.4 -	3.5-4.9 < 500 ml/d	> 5.0 < 200 ml/d

DEFINITION

Neonatal sepsis is a clinical syndrome in the first 28 days from birth manifested by systemic signs of infection and isolation of a bacterial pathogen from the bloodstream. A consensus definition for neonatal sepsis is lacking.

DIAGNOSTIC CRITERIA

The diagnosis of neonatal sepsis is based on the provider's assessment of many factors including clinical presentation, blood cultures, identification of an infection, nonspecific markers of sepsis (including C-reactive protein and procalcitonin), and biomolecular testing including PCR (DNA polymerase chain reaction).

Some important diagnostic indicators include:

- Temperature > 100.4° F/> 38.0° C lasting > 1 hour associated with infection; or < 97.7° F/< 36.5° C
- Poor general appearance and behavior (decreased activity, irritability, lethargy, hypotonia, poor nursing/feeding)
- Respiratory difficulty such as tachypnea (> 40; > 50 for 0-7 days old), weak respiratory effort, hypoxemia, grunting, irregular breathing, episodes of apnea
- Tachycardia (> 160) or bradycardia (< 100)
- WBC > 34,000 for 0-7 days; > 19,500 or < 5000 for 8-28 days
- Systolic BP < 65
- Cutaneous: pale or marbled with petechiae or purple, mottling, cold skin, cyanosis, jaundice

High risk factors include:

- Apgar ≤ 6
- Low birth weight/prematurity
- Maternal perinatal infection, colonization, or fever
- Prolonged maternal rupture of membranes
- Meconium stained amniotic fluid (MSAF)

- Inadequate prenatal care
- Invasive procedure

The main causative organisms are Staph, Strep, enterococcus, gram-negatives, anaerobes, and occasionally Listeria.

CODING AND DOCUMENTATION CHALLENGES

Neonatal sepsis is assigned to category P36 (Bacterial sepsis in the newborn) which includes both congenital (in utero) and acquired cases.

Category P36 includes specific codes for Staph, Strep, E. coli, and anaerobes. If the organism is unspecified, assign code P36.9.

If applicable, assign an additional code for severe sepsis (R65.20 or R65.21) and any associated acute organ dysfunction.

Suspected sepsis. A common practice is routinely giving IV antibiotics to many neonates lasting 2-3 days until cultures are negative on the premise that neonatal sepsis may be difficult to detect. Providers may document a diagnosis of "suspected sepsis" that is subsequently ruled out. In this case, do not assign code P36.9 (neonatal sepsis) unless sepsis remains suspected or is confirmed and a full course of antibiotics administered. Instead assign code Z05.1, Newborn affected by maternal infectious and parasitic diseases.

References

- Official Coding Guidelines I.C.16.f
- Early-Onset Neonatal Sepsis: Clin Microbiol Rev 2014; 27 p. 21–47
- InTech Publishing: Neonatal Bacterial Infection. Chapter 1—Early Detection and Prevention of Neonatal Sepsis
- UpToDate.com: Clinical features, evaluation and diagnosis in term and late preterm infant
- Coding Clinic 2016 Fourth Quarter p. 76
- Coding Clinic 2019 Second Quarter p. 10.

DEFINITION

Pediatric SIRS in the presence of, or as a result of, suspected or proven infection. The clinical criteria for pediatric sepsis/SIRS are quite different from the adult criteria and also depend upon the age of the patient. Viral sepsis is a common cause of fever requiring admission when bacterial sepsis is ruled out.

DIAGNOSTIC CRITERIA

Two or more (one must be temperature or WBC) of the following:

- Core temperature (oral, rectal) > 101.3° F/> 38.5° C or < 96.8° F/< 36.0° C
- WBC elevated or depressed for age (not due to chemotherapy) or > 10% bands
- Tachycardia: Heart rate > 2 SD above normal for age not due to other stimuli
- Tachypnea: Respiratory rate > 2 SD above normal for age, or mechanical ventilation (not due to anesthesia or neuromuscular disease)
- Bradycardia (≤ 1 year): Heart rate < 10th percentile for age not due to other specific causes.

Age	Heart Rate	Resp Rate	WBC
29 days–1 year	> 180	> 34	> 17.5 or < 5
1–2 years	> 160	> 26	> 15.5 or < 6
2–5 years	> 140	> 22	> 15.5 or < 6
6–11 years	> 130	> 20	> 13.5 or < 4.5
12 –18 years	> 110	> 20	> 12 or < 4.5

The above indicators for vital signs and WBC are rough approximations and vary by source. Individual institutions may have established their own criteria.

Note significant differences between 2005 International Pediatric Consensus Conference Definitions (especially ages 13 to < 18) and adult Sepsis-2 SIRS criteria (beginning age 18) for tachycardia, respiratory rate, and WBC.

Severe Sepsis. Sepsis with acute organ dysfunction, hypoperfusion or hypotension. May include: hypoxemia, respiratory failure, hypotension, mental status changes/encephalopathy, coagulopathy, liver failure, acute renal failure.

Septic Shock. For pediatric criteria for shock, see *Shock*.

CODING AND DOCUMENTATION CHALLENGES

Sepsis-3 criteria apply only to adults.

An update to the Pediatric Sepsis management guidelines was published in 2020 which maintained the 2005 Pediatric sepsis consensus definition and criteria. A revision of the 2005 consensus definition and criteria are expected but remain pending at this time.

References

- International Pediatric Sepsis Consensus Conference: Definitions for sepsis and organ dysfunction in pediatrics. Pediatr Crit Care Med 2005; 6: 2–8
- Surviving Sepsis Campaign International Guidelines for the Management of Septic Shock and Sepsis-Associated Organ Dysfunction in Children. Pediatr Crit Care Med 2020; 21: e52-e106
- UpToDate.com: Bradycardia in Children
- E-Medicine Health: Pediatric Vital Signs
- ICD-10-CM Official Coding Guidelines Section I.C.1.d.

DEFINITION

A pathophysiologic state of generalized inadequate tissue perfusion causing cellular hypoxia (decreased oxygen delivery to tissues) and usually associated with profound hypotension. Shock may result from trauma, blood loss, severe infection, acute MI, allergic reaction, poisoning, heatstroke, severe burns, or other causes.

Components of shock may include:
- Reduced cardiac output (CO)
- Peripheral vasoconstriction (increased systemic vascular resistance—SVR) causing tissue hypoxia
- Peripheral vasodilation (decreased SVR) exceeding cardiac capacity to maintain blood pressure and tissue perfusion
- Inadequate blood volume with insufficient oxygen delivery

DIAGNOSTIC CRITERIA (ADULT)

- Hypotension refractory to effective fluid resuscitation (40ml/kg over one hour):
  - Systolic blood pressure (SBP) < 90 mmHg, or
  - Mean arterial pressure (MAP) < 70 mmHg, or
  - Decrease baseline SBP of ≥ 40 mmHg

- Lactate level > 4 mmol/L is equivalent to shock without BP parameters.

Note: MAP has traditionally been measured by intra-arterial monitoring. As an alternative approximation, many current external blood pressure monitors now have MAP calculating technology.

DIAGNOSTIC CRITERIA (PEDIATRIC)

- Age 0–28 days = SBP < 60 mmHg
- Age 1–12 mos = SBP < 70 mmHg
- Age 1–9 yrs = SBP < 70 mmHg + 2x age
- Age ≥ 10 yrs = SBP < 90 mmHg
- Lactic acidosis (any age)

TREATMENT

Treatment includes IV fluid resuscitation and/or blood transfusion, correction of underlying cause, supplemental oxygen, or vasopressor infusion such as norepinephrine or dopamine.

CODING AND DOCUMENTATION CHALLENGES

Documentation of the cause or type of shock should be obtained.

R57.9	Shock unspecified	CC
T81.10XA*	Shock during or resulting from a procedure	CC
T81.11XA T81.12XA T81.19XA	Cardiogenic shock, postprocedural Septic shock, postprocedural Hypovolemic or other shock, postprocedural	MCC MCC MCC
R57.0	Cardiogenic: Inadequate cardiac output	MCC
R57.1	Hypovolemic: Depletion of intravascular volume	MCC
R57.8	Hemorrhagic or other specified	MCC
T79.4XXA	Post-traumatic or traumatic: typically due to hemorrhage or severe SIRS	MCC
R65.21	Septic: Includes endotoxic and gram-negative	MCC
A48.3	Toxic shock: Toxin-producing staph aureus (50% menstrual related)	MCC

*Do not assign codes for postprocedural shock unless it occurs during surgery or specified as resulting from the procedure by a provider.

Codes R57.9, R57.0, R57.1, and R57.8 are symptom codes, and the cause, if known, is sequenced first.

References

- UpToDate.com: Definition, classification, etiology, and pathophysiology of shock in adults
- UpToDate.com: Initial evaluation of shock in the adult trauma patient and management of non-hemorrhagic shock
- UpToDate.com: Initial management of shock in children
- UpToDate.com: Staphylococcal toxic shock syndrome.

DEFINITION

SIRS due to causes other than infection. Causes may include pancreatitis, trauma, malignancies, bowel infarction, extensive burns, major surgical procedures, tumor lysis syndrome, and cytokine release syndrome.

DIAGNOSTIC CRITERIA

SIRS is defined by the Sepsis-2 criteria which are identical for both infectious and non-infectious SIRS. See *Sepsis-2* diagnostic criteria.

CODING AND DOCUMENTATION CHALLENGES

Physicians, even those who are familiar with the definition of non-infectious SIRS, may forget to document it. A query for clarification is often needed.

For non-infectious SIRS, the underlying condition causing it is sequenced first, followed by the appropriate SIRS code. These codes cannot be assigned as principal diagnosis.

- R65.10 without acute organ dysfunction (CC)
- R65.11 with acute organ dysfunction (MCC)

According to OCG I.C.18.g, "If acute organ dysfunction is documented, but it cannot be determined if the acute organ dysfunction is associated with SIRS or due to another condition (e.g., directly due to the trauma), the provider should be queried."

If shock is documented, an additional code for the type of shock is also assigned.

References
- Same as Sepsis-2
- Official Coding Guidelines I.C.18.g and I.C.1.d.6
- Coding Clinic 2014 Third Quarter p. 4.

DEFINITION

Non-Pressure Ulcers. Non-pressure, chronic ulcers are defined as erosion of the epidermis or dermis but can extend to the subcutaneous fat, fascia, muscle, ligaments, tendons, and bone, and generally caused by poor blood flow. Chronic is defined as lasting three months or more.

Common causes of skin ulcers include diabetes (ischemic and non-ischemic), ischemia (peripheral artery disease), neuropathy, venous insufficiency (stasis), infection, vasculitis, and trauma.

The great majority of non-pressure ulcers are located in the lower extremities. Likewise, almost all lower extremity ulcers are non-pressure in nature, except heel ulcers which are almost always due to pressure. Non-pressure ulcers are classified based on depth.

Patients with skin ulcers, especially of the lower legs, have a high risk of developing **cellulitis**. Cellulitis is a bacterial infection of the skin. Symptoms of cellulitis include swelling, redness, and can be painful and tender to touch.

Pressure Ulcers. In contrast, pressure ulcers are defined as localized damage to the skin and/or underlying soft tissue due to intense or prolonged pressure often associated with immobility and/or absent sensation. Moisture and nutritional deficiency (or obesity) also contribute.

Common locations for pressure ulcers include sacrum/coccyx, heel, buttocks (gluteal), hip, low back, elbow. Most foot/ankle ulcers other than heel are not pressure ulcers.

Only pressure ulcers are staged; others may be classified based on depth.

DIAGNOSTIC CRITERIA—PRESSURE ULCERS

Stage 1 - *Non-blanching erythema of intact skin:* Normal skin turns pale (blanches) when pressed with a finger then returns promptly to normal color because blood is squeezed out of capillaries by the pressure and quickly refills when pressure released (may appear differently in darkly pigmented skin).

In Stage 1 pressure ulcer, pressing with a finger does not blanch because there has been capillary damage and microscopic skin hemorrhage that cannot be pressed out.

Stage 2 - *Partial thickness (epidermal) skin loss* exposing the vascular dermis (like a superficial abrasion). The wound bed is viable, pink or red, moist; may also present as an intact or ruptured serum-filled blister. Subcutaneous adipose tissue (fat) and deeper tissues are not exposed.

Stage 3 - *Full thickness skin loss (MCC):* Full-thickness loss of skin, in which subcutaneous adipose tissue is exposed and visible in the ulcer; granulation tissue (microscopic connective tissue and blood vessels that have a granular appearance) is often present. Fascia, muscle, tendon, ligament, cartilage and/or bone are not exposed.

Stage 4 - *Full-thickness skin and tissue loss (MCC):* Full-thickness skin and tissue loss with exposed or directly palpable fascia, muscle, tendon, ligament, cartilage or bone in the ulcer.

Deep tissue pressure injury *(DTPI)* - Intact or non-intact skin with localized area of persistent non-blanchable deep red, maroon, purple discoloration or epidermal separation revealing a dark wound bed or blood-filled blister.

Unstageable - *Obscured full-thickness and tissue loss*: Full-thickness skin and tissue loss in which the extent of tissue damage within the ulcer cannot be confirmed because it is obscured by slough or eschar. If slough or eschar is removed, a Stage 3 or 4 pressure injury will be revealed.

Unspecified - Do not confuse "unstageable" (L89.--0) with "unspecified" (L89.--9), which is assigned when there is no documentation regarding stage. All pressure ulcers should be staged or classified as noted above.

TREATMENT

Wound care/dressings, debridement, other more extensive surgical intervention, wound care referral for management, hyperbaric oxygen.

Initiation or adjustment of pain medication, antibiotics, application of topicals, other medication related to the ulcer.

The treatment of advanced stages is individualized according to extent, nature, severity, and complications, including excision and debridement of devitalized/necrotic tissue; wet-to-dry saline or hypochlorite solution packing/dressings; topical antibiotics; specialized gels.

CODING AND DOCUMENTATION CHALLENGES

ICD-10 classifies chronic (present for > 3 months) non-pressure ulcers according to location and depth. Depth is classified as skin breakdown only, exposure of subcutaneous fat, necrosis of muscle, necrosis of bone, or unspecified. Acute, transient, or reversible ulcers due to such things as minor trauma, spider bites, and resolved infections should not be assigned to these codes.

Patients admitted with skin ulcers often have evidence of **cellulitis**. Sequencing depends upon the focus of admission or may be co-equal. Cellulitis can usually be treated initially on an outpatient basis unless sepsis or another complication is present or failed outpatient treatment necessitates inpatient admission. Cellulitis is unlikely to be the principal diagnosis if excisional debridement is performed. Look also for evidence of "**necrotic**" tissue which is coded to gangrene, code I96, if not elsewhere classified; e.g., if with diabetes is coded to E11.52.

Pressure ulcers are also described as "pressure injury" to emphasize that both intact and ulcerated skin may be involved.

Documentation. Pressure ulcers are classified as combination codes assigned by stage and location. The provider must document the presence, location, and POA status of pressure ulcers. A non-physician healthcare professional (e.g., nurse) may document the stage.

Stages 3 & 4 pressure ulcers are MCCs and CMS-HCCs 157 & 158. All stage 3 & 4 pressure ulcers (including Kennedy ulcers), unstageable, and DTPI are included in PSI-3 if not present on admission.

Unstageable pressure ulcers are commonly stage 3 or 4, so providers may be able to clarify that they are probably or suspected to be Stage 3 or 4.

Deep tissue pressure injury (DTPI), by definition "deep tissue" can be inferred clinically as Stage 3 or 4, but not for code assignment. Different codes are used to specifically identify deep tissue injury or deep tissue pressure injury, codes L89.--6, which are non-CCs.

If after debridement of the DTPI or unstageable pressure ulcer the stage is revealed, assign the code for the pressure ulcer and the stage only.

According to OCG, if a patient is admitted with a pressure ulcer at one stage and it **progresses to a higher stage,** assign one code for that site and ulcer stage on admission (POA=Y) and a second code for the same ulcer site and the highest stage reported during the stay (POA=N).

Healing/healed pressure ulcer. Pressure ulcers described as "healing" should be assigned the appropriate stage code based on the documentation in the medical record. If documented as "healed" at the time of admission, no code is assigned. For ulcers that were present on admission but healed at the time of discharge, assign the code for the site and stage for the pressure ulcer at the time of admission (OCG section I.C.12.a.5).

For **DRG Tips**, see DRG 592-594, Skin ulcers.

References

- Revised National Pressure Ulcer Advisory Panel Pressure Injury Staging System 2016
- UpToDate.com: Clinical assessment of chronic wounds
- UpToDate.com: Approach to the differential diagnosis of leg ulcers
- Coding Clinic 2016 Third Quarter p. 38
- Coding Clinic 2021 First Quarter p. 24
- UpToDate.com: Clinical staging and management of pressure-induced skin and soft tissue injury
- UpToDate.com: Epidemiology, pathogenesis, and risk assessment of pressure-induced skin and soft tissue ulcers
- Official Coding Guidelines I.C.12.a. and Appendix I: POA Reporting Guidelines.

DEFINITION

The American Psychiatric Association's Diagnostic and Statistical Manual of Mental Disorders (DSM-5) is the official source for diagnostic criteria of mental disorders and substance-related disorders.

Substances include alcohol, cannabis, hallucinogens, inhalants, opioids (e.g., heroin), sedatives, hypnotics, or anxiolytics (e.g., valium, "quaaludes"), and stimulants (cocaine, methamphetamine), among others.

Alcohol use disorder requires a problematic pattern of alcohol use leading to clinically significant impairment or distress. It does not include simple alcohol use that is not problematic.

Drug use disorder is a problematic pattern of drug use leading to clinically significant impairment or distress.

Nonprescription use of a drug should be clinically considered problematic abuse/dependence, and DSM-5 identifies any use of illicit drugs (like heroin, cocaine, methamphetamine, etc.) as problematic.

Remission ("in remission") is prior alcohol or drug dependence with current abstinence.

The diagnosis of a substance (alcohol or drug) use disorder is based upon a set of problematic behaviors related to the use of that substance. These behaviors include impaired control, social impairment, risky use, tolerance, and withdrawal as outlined below.

DIAGNOSTIC CRITERIA

There are 11 different DSM-5 clinical criteria for substance-related disorders which include:

1. Using larger amounts/longer
2. Repeated attempts to quit/control use
3. Much time spent getting, using, or recovering from the drug use
4. Craving: Strong desire or urge to use the substance

5. Neglecting major roles due to use
6. Social/interpersonal problems related to use
7. Activities given up because of use
8. Hazardous use: repeatedly using substances in physically dangerous situations
9. Physical/psychological problems related to use
10. Tolerance: Need to increase the amount of a substance to achieve the same desired effect
11. Withdrawal: Cessation of use results in a cluster of very unpleasant symptoms; substance is taken to relieve or avoid withdrawal symptoms.

DSM-5 uses the terms mild, moderate, and severe to classify the substance use disorder. Severity is determined by the number of diagnostic criteria applicable to each patient:

- Mild = 2-3 criteria
- Moderate = 4-5 criteria
- Severe = 6 or more criteria

Substance withdrawal. Withdrawal syndrome almost always occurs when individuals who are substance dependent abruptly discontinue it. However, even in regular use or abuse of substances, withdrawal can occur.

Alcohol withdrawal symptoms typically begin within six hours of the last drink and tend to spike around 24 to 72 hours. Withdrawal symptoms include anxiety, agitation, restlessness, insomnia, tremor, palpitations, headache, alcohol craving, diaphoresis, loss of appetite, nausea and vomiting. Treatment may include valium, ativan, librium, and alcohol abstinence counseling.

Opioid use. Patients who require multiple daily doses (2-3 or more) for more than two to four weeks are highly likely to become dependent and sometimes begin to show evidence of tolerance.

If a withdrawal syndrome has not actually occurred but it is likely to occur if discontinued, this situation in itself would not be considered a substance use disorder.

For patients who are therapeutically opioid-dependent, providers should be making repeated periodic attempts over time to reduce doses or wean patients off of opioids, supporting them with non-opioid pain medications or with less potent opioids.

Patients who take opioids on a prn basis, only once or twice a day or not every day, are unlikely to develop problematic patterns, experience withdrawal if discontinued, or develop tolerance. Symptoms of opioid withdrawal include anxiety, nausea, vomiting, or abdominal pain.

The ultimate decision of what constitutes use, abuse, and dependence is determined by the physician's clinical judgment.

CODING AND DOCUMENTATION CHALLENGES

Drug dependence (e.g., opioids, cocaine, heroin, benzodiazepines, stimulants) and alcohol/drug use, abuse, or dependence with a specified "substance-induced disorder" are CCs.

In addition, substance use or abuse (in addition to dependence) with withdrawal are also CCs. For example, alcohol use or abuse with withdrawal (F10.930 or F10.130), opioid abuse with withdrawal (F11.13), cocaine abuse or use with withdrawal (F14.13, F14.93), other stimulant abuse with withdrawal (F15.13).

Dependence. The 11 DSM-5 diagnostic criteria for substance use disorders (see above) can be used to determine if the substance use is mild, moderate, or severe.

A substance use disorder documented as moderate (4-5 criteria) or severe (6+ criteria) is classified in ICD-10 as "dependence" and is coded F10.20 for alcohol or F11.20 for opioid. Mild substance use disorder (2-3 criteria) is classified as "abuse."

Withdrawal. According to Coding Clinic 2020 Fourth Quarter p. 17, "Substance withdrawal can occur in clinical situations involving individuals who do not have a diagnosis of substance dependence but use substances regularly and then suddenly stop using them."

It is common for patients with problematic drug or alcohol use to experience withdrawal symptoms while in the hospital. Review the progress or nursing notes for withdrawal symptoms. Use of a drug or alcohol withdrawal assessment scale (e.g., COWS, CIWA, WAS) may also identify withdrawal symptoms and confirm withdrawal based on a point system.

Alcohol withdrawal symptoms often develop when a patient still has a high blood alcohol level, although lack of a positive alcohol blood test does not negate the diagnosis of alcohol use or abuse or withdrawal symptoms. Since alcohol is eliminated from the blood stream in approximately 12 hours, it may not be detected in an alcohol blood test.

Substance-induced disorders. The codes for unspecified substance use with a substance-induced disorder is included in codes F10.9-, F11.9-, F12.9-, F13.9-, F14.9-, F15.9-, F16.9-, F18.9-, F19.9-. For example, F10.9- includes alcohol use with intoxication, withdrawal, and other "alcohol-induced" mental or behavioral disorders. These codes are to be used only when the substance use is associated with a specific substance-related disorder or medical condition, and such a relationship is documented by the provider.

Medical conditions due to substance use, abuse, and dependence (e.g., alcoholic liver failure or alcoholic pancreatitis) are not classified as substance-induced disorders. For example, alcoholic acute pancreatitis due to alcohol dependence, would be assigned code K70.40, Alcoholic liver failure, and code F10.20, Alcohol dependence, uncomplicated. It would not be appropriate to assign code F10.288, Alcohol dependence with other alcohol-induced disorder (see OCG Section I.C.5.b.4).

Note that intoxication or withdrawal must be present during the visit (not just a "history of") to be assigned.

Do not confuse these ICD-10 defined "substance-induced" disorders with the 11 DSM-5 criteria that define "substance use" disorders and their severity. It is important to distinguish between the coexistence of a non-induced condition versus a condition that is specifically induced by alcohol or drugs, which is usually a professional clinical judgment.

Recognizing, documenting, and addressing these disorders are challenging since physicians may not recognize, document, or address them.

Opioid use. Per Coding Clinic 2018 Second Quarter, p. 11, patients taking opioids for chronic pain as prescribed by the physician and without an associated physical, behavioral, or mental disorder should not be coded as "opioid use." For opioid use including maintenance therapy that is not problematic, i.e., no identified substance-induced disorder, ICD-10 indicates that the correct code is "long term (current) use of opiate analgesic" (code Z79.891).

Providers should not use the term "**alcoholism**" anymore because it is not recognized by DSM-5, results in assignment of F10.20 (dependence) when abuse should be used, and labels the patient as "dependent." The alcohol use disorder (use, abuse, dependence) codes are not to be used for patients who drink moderately with no problematic consequences.

CMS-HCCs 54 and 55 includes drug dependence; alcohol/drug use, abuse, or dependence with a specified substance-induced disorder; alcohol dependence; and alcohol and drug dependence, in remission.

References

- UpToDate.com: Clinical assessment of substance use disorders
- UpToDate.com: Risky drinking and alcohol use disorder: Epidemiology, pathogenesis, clinical manifestations, course, assessment, and diagnosis
- UpToDate.com: Approach to treating alcohol use disorder
- UpToDate.com: Alcohol withdrawal: Epidemiology, clinical manifestations, course, assessment, and diagnosis
- The American Psychiatric Association's Diagnostic and Statistical Manual of Mental Disorders (DSM-5)
- Coding Clinic 2018 Second Quarter p. 11
- Coding Clinic 2020 Fourth Quarter p. 16-17.

DEFINITION

Transbronchial biopsy crosses the bronchial wall to obtain tissue from the lung. It is often used to diagnose lung neoplasm, interstitial fibrosis, sarcoidosis, or unexplained pulmonary infection or infiltrate.

CODING AND DOCUMENTATION CHALLENGES

Transbronchial biopsy uses the root operation "**excision**" by specific site and is considered a surgical procedure that impacts DRG assignment. *Example*: Transbronchial biopsy (excision) of left lower lobe of lung, endoscopic, diagnostic (code 0BBJ8ZX).

A code for transbronchial biopsy is assigned if documented as "transbronchial" or the target is identified as lung (not bronchus). Review the procedure note carefully for evidence of transbronchial biopsy of a lung target.

Lung tissue (alveoli) on the pathology report supports assignment of transbronchial biopsy. However, the absence of lung tissue in the pathology report does not preclude the assignment of a transbronchial biopsy when the procedure is performed and documented as such by the provider. Lung tissue samples may be inadequate, inconclusive, or show nothing but the pathologic condition (such as lung cancer) that has completely replaced lung tissue in the sample.

Transbronchial needle aspiration (TBNA), transbronchial cryobiopsy, or fine needle aspiration to obtain an aspirated sample of lung, lymph node or endobronchial lesion use the root operation "**extraction**" by specific site and are not O.R. procedures that impact DRG assignment.

Bronchial or endobronchial biopsies, bronchoalveolar lavage (BAL), including bronchial brushing and washing to obtain endobronchial material, are considered minor endoscopic procedures that do not impact DRG assignment.

References
- Coding Clinic 2016 First Quarter p. 26
- UpToDate.com: Flexible bronchoscopy in adults.

DEFINITION

A TIA is a temporary blockage of blood flow to the brain. It produces similar symptoms as a CVA but usually do not last very long and cause no permanent damage. Often called a "mini-stroke." Typical neurologic deficits include focal weakness, impaired speech, difficulty with balance or walking.

DIAGNOSTIC CRITERIA

TIA is defined by both:

- Transient focal neurological deficit lasting < 24 hours, and
- No acute infarction or hemorrhage on imaging

Duration is counted from onset, not presentation. Patients often present having already had symptoms for several hours or more.

Persistence of a focal neurological deficit > 24 hours from onset is a stroke (CVA), not TIA, even with negative imaging.

While the duration of symptoms required to establish a diagnosis of TIA officially remains < 24 hours, it is a subject of debate among neurologists with many experts suggesting it should only be one hour. About one-third of patients with stroke symptoms for < 24 hours have a positive lesion of MRI.

Causes of TIA include:

- **Cerebral/pre-cerebral stenosis**: Any degree of stenosis may cause a TIA. "Non-critical stenosis" indicates that medical therapy is preferred to surgery; it does not exclude stenosis as the cause.

- **Transient cerebral embolism** due to platelet aggregates is often caused by atrial fibrillation, abnormal heart valves, or atrial septal defect (ASD).

- **Vertebrobasilar syndrome** is considered nothing more than a TIA symptom, but documentation of stenosis, occlusion, thrombosis, embolism of any vertebrobasilar arteries is a serious cause.

Common sources of transient cerebral embolism include:

- Atrial fibrillation—especially if PT/INR is subtherapeutic
- Valvular heart disease (aortic or mitral valves)
- ASD with "paradoxical embolus" of small clots from the right (venous) side of the heart across the ASD to the left heart and from there up to the brain
- Mural (ventricular wall) thrombus—especially following MI
- Any degree of stenosis/narrowing of a carotid, vertebral or cerebral artery

Diagnostic testing often includes trans-esophageal echocardiogram (TEE), carotid or transcranial Doppler, CT, MRI, and MRA—all looking for sources of emboli, stenosis, occlusion, or thrombosis.

TREATMENT

Treatment includes anti-platelet therapy, such as aspirin, Persantin, Aggrenox, or Plavix, to prevent recurrent thrombosis or embolism, even when no significant abnormality is identified. Less often, an anti-coagulant like Coumadin may be prescribed.

CODING AND DOCUMENTATION CHALLENGES

TIA is actually a symptom of a significant underlying cerebrovascular process. It's the underlying condition that really matters and is treated, not the symptom.

Even if nothing is found on evaluation to explain the TIA, the most likely cause of TIA is unexplained "transient cerebral embolism."

For **DRG Tips**, see DRG 69, Transient ischemia.

References

- National Stroke Association Guidelines for the Management of Transient Ischemic Attacks. Ann Neurol 2006; 60: 301–313
- Diagnosis and Management of Transient Ischemic Attack, National Library of Medicine 2017
- Acute Stroke (Cerebrovascular Accident). National Library of Medicine: Stat Pearls NBK535369
- UpToDate.com: Initial evaluation and management of transient ischemic attack and minor ischemic stroke.

Diagnosis	Results / Indicators
AKI	• Creatinine increase ≥ 1.5 x baseline • Creatinine increase ≥ 0.3 *within 48 hours*
Alcohol Withdrawal	CIWA: < 8 no withdrawal, 8-10 mild, 10-15 moderate, > 15 severe withdrawal
CKD	Stage 3a: GFR 45-59, Stage 3b: GFR 30-44, Stage 4: GFR 15-29, Stage 5: GFR < 15, ESRD - on chronic dialysis
Functional Quadriplegia	Braden Scores: • Mobility = 1 (completely immobile) or 2 (very limited) • Activity = 1 (bedridden)
Hypertensive crisis	Crisis: SBP > 180, or DPB > 120 Emergency: with end organ dysfunction Urgency: w/o end organ dysfunction
Intellectual Disability	IQ range: 20-35 (severe); < 20 (profound)
Metabolic acidosis	Bicarb ($HCO3$) < 22 and/or chloride > 106
Metabolic alkalosis	Bicarb ($HCO3$) > 28
Neonatal Abstinence Syndrome	Withdrawal is a score of ≥ 8 at two consecutive measurements
Opiate Withdrawal (COWS)	5-12 mild, 13-24 moderate, 25-36 moderately severe, > 36 severe withdrawal
Pancytopenia	• Neutropenia: ANC < 1.8 k • Thrombocytopenia: Platelets < 150 k • Anemia: Hgb < 13.0 (men), < 12.0 (women)
Postnatal depression	Finnegan screening: ≥ 10 is possible depression
Respiratory acidosis	pH < 7.35 + $pCO2$ > 45
Respiratory alkalosis	pH > 7.45+ $pCO2$ < 35
Respiratory failure	Hypoxemic: $pO2$ < 60 or $SpO2$ < 91% on RA Hypercapnic: $CO2$ > 50 + pH < 7.35 (if acute) P/F Ratio*: ABG: $PaO2$ ($pO2$) / $FIO2$ < 300 Ex. $pO2$ = 65 / 0.32 (3 L/min) = 203 *Do not use for chronic resp failure pts on home O2*

Diagnosis	Results / Indicators

OVERVIEW

This section provides a list of common or important comorbid conditions that are MCC, CC, or HCC with the APR-DRG standard severity of illness (SOI) subclass. Also included is the CMS-HCC V24.0 listing.

Comorbid conditions that are an MCC are indicated in bold. Those conditions that are not MCC or CC but are an HCC are *italicized*. Approximately half of all HCCs are not MCC/CC and although not impacting DRG assignment, they are primarily chronic conditions and may contribute to risk adjustment.

There are many diagnoses included in each MCC, CC, or HCC category, but the examples listed are the least specific or severe although the more specific or severe codes would also be included.

Clinical indicators for many of these comorbid conditions are covered in detail in the **Key References** section of this guide. The coding of a specific diagnosis should be evaluated on a case-by-case basis and based on physician documentation in the medical record.

Always remember that in order to code a comorbid condition as a secondary diagnosis, it must first meet the definition of a secondary diagnosis. The definition of a secondary diagnosis is an additional condition (either present on admission or occurring during admission) that requires any of the following:

- Clinical evaluation, or
- Therapeutic treatment, or
- Diagnostic procedures, or
- Increased nursing care/monitoring, or
- Extended length of stay

A complete listing of the FY2022 MCCs and CCs and the CMS-HCC V24.0 ICD-10 codes are available at *www.pinsonandtang.com*.

Comorbid Conditions
MCC in bold

CC non-bold

Non-CC/MCC in italics
(HCC and/or SOI only)

ICD-10 *Codes listed do not include all codes available for the diagnosis, only the least specific code to meet the MCC/CC status.*

HCC *CMS-HCC #. See CMS-HCC List that follows for HCC description and weight.*

SOI *Standard SOI subclass for APR-DRGs.*

Comorbid Conditions	ICD-10	HCC	SOI
Abdominal aortic aneurysm (AAA)	*I714*	*108*	*-*
Acidosis: metabolic/respiratory/lactic	E872	-	2
Alkalosis: metabolic/respiratory	E873	-	2
Acute coronary insufficiency	I248	87	2
Acute coronary thrombosis/embolism (not resulting in MI)	I240	87	2
Acute coronary syndrome (ACS)	I249	87	2
Acute kidney injury (AKI)	N179	135	2
Acute tubular necrosis (ATN)	N170	135	**4**
Adult respiratory distress syndrome (ARDS)	J80	84	2
Alcohol dependence	*F1020*	*55*	*-*
Alcohol dependence, in remission	*F1021*	*55*	*-*
Alcohol use or abuse with withdrawal	F10.130	55	-
Alcohol use with alcohol-use disorder	F1099	55	2
Alcoholic liver disease	*K709*	*28*	*-*
Amputation status, lower limb: toes, foot, ankle, below or above knee	*Z89411-Z89619*	*189*	*-*
Anemia, acute blood loss (ABLA)	D62	-	2
Anemia in CKD	*D631*	*-*	*2*
Aneurysm	*I729*	*108*	*-*
Angina	*I209*	*88*	*-*
Angina, unstable	I200	87	2
Aortic aneurysm	*I719*	*108*	*-*
Aortic atherosclerosis	*I700*	*108*	*-*
Aplastic anemia	D619	46	3
Artificial opening status	*Z939*	*188*	*-*

Comorbid Conditions	ICD-10	HCC	SOI
Atelectasis	J9811	-	-
Atrial fibrillation, unspecified	*I4891*	*96*	*-*
Atrial fibrillation, chronic	I4820	96	2
Atrial fibrillation, permanent	I4821	96	2
Atrial flutter	I4892	96	2
Atrial septal defect (ASD)	Q211	-	-
Avascular necrosis (AVN)	M879	39	2
Bacteremia	R7881	-	3
Bipolar disorder	*F319*	*59*	*-*
Bleeding, GI	K922	-	2
Bleeding, rectal/anal	K625	-	-
Blood in stool (melena)	K921	-	-
BMI ≤ 19.9	Z681	-	-
BMI ≥ 40	Z6841	22	-
Brain compression/herniation	G935	80	2
Brain death	G9382	-	**4**
Bronchiectasis	*J479*	*112*	*-*
Bronchitis, chronic	*J42*	*111*	*-*
Cachexia (cachetic)	R64	21	2
CAD of bypass graft	I25810	-	2
Cancer, lung	C3490	9	-
Carcinomatosis	C800	8	2
Cardiac arrest (dc'd alive)	I469	84	**-**
Cardiomyopathy, unspecified	I429	85	2
Cellulitis	L0390	-	-
Cellulitis, leg	L03119	-	-
Cerebral edema	G936	80	**4**
Cerebral palsy: spastic quadriplegic	G800	74	2
Cerebral palsy: athetoid, ataxic, spastic	G801-G803	74	2
Cerebrovascular accident (CVA)	I6350	100	**4**
Cerebral hemorrhage	I619	99	**4**
CHF, unspecified	*I509*	*85*	*-*

Comorbid Conditions	ICD-10	HCC	SOI
Cirrhosis of liver	*K7460*	*28*	*-*
CKD, Stage 3	*N1830*	*138*	*-*
CKD, Stage 4	N184	137	-
CKD, Stage 5	N185	136	-
CKD, Stage 5, on dialysis (ESRD)	N186	136	2
Clostridium difficle (c.diff) colitis	A0472	-	3
Cocaine use or abuse with withdrawal	F1493	55	-
Colostomy status	*Z933*	*188*	*-*
Coma	R4020	80	**4**
COPD, acute exacerbation (AECOPD)	J441	111	2
COPD, with acute bronchitis	J440	111	2
COPD, unspecified	*J449*	*111*	*2*
Cor pulmonale	*I2781*	*85*	*2*
Cor pulmonale, acute w/ PE	I2609	85	**4**
COVID-19	U07.1	-	3
Crohn's disease	K5090	35	-
CSF (cerebrospinal fluid) leak	G9600	-	2
Cystic fibrosis	E849	110	2
Cytokine release syndrome, Grade 3-5	D89833	-	2
Deep vein thrombosis (DVT)	I8291	-	3
Delirium, drug-induced	F19921	55	2
Demand ischemia	I248	87	2
Dementia, with behavioral disturbance	F0391	51	2
Depression, major: mild, moderate, recurrent	F320, F321, F339	59	2
Depression, major, in remission	F3340	59	-
Diabetes mellitus (any type)	*E119*	*19*	*-*
Diabetes with any related complication: nephropathy, neuropathy, etc.	*E1121-E118*	*18*	*-*
Diabetes with hyperglycemia	*E1165*	*18*	*-*
Diabetes, hyperosmolar (Type II)	E1100	17	3
Diabetes, with hypoglycemia & coma	E11641	17	**4**

Comorbid Conditions	ICD-10	HCC	SOI
Diabetes, with ketoacidosis (Type II)	E1110	17	3
Diverticulosis with bleeding	K5791	-	3
Drug dependence (hallucinogens, inhalants, opioid, sedatives, hypnotics, anxiolytics, stimulants)	F1120, F1320. . . F1920	55	- 2 -
Drug dependence, in remission	*F1921*	*55*	*-*
Emaciation [cachexia]	R64	21	2
Emphysema	*J439*	*111*	*-*
Encephalopathy	G9340	-	3
Encephalopathy, alcoholic	F1027	54	2
Encephalopathy, anoxic, hypoxic	G931	80	2
Encephalopathy, chronic static	G9349	-	3
Encephalopathy, hypertensive	I674	-	3
Encephalopathy, metabolic	G9341	-	3
Encephalopathy, toxic	G92.9	-	3
Enteritis, bacterial	A049	-	2
Enteritis, E. coli	A044	-	2
Esophageal erosions or ulcer	K2210	-	2
Esophageal ulcer with bleeding	K2211	-	3
Esophagitis, candida	B3781	6	2
Esophagitis with bleeding	K20.91	-	2
ESRD	N186	136	2
Functional quadriplegia	R532	70	3
Gastritis, hemorrhagic	K2971	-	3
GERD with esophagitis with bleeding	K21.01	-	2
GI bleeding	K922	-	2
Hallucinations	R443	-	-
Heart failure, unspecified	*I509*	*85*	*-*
Heart failure, diastolic	I5030	85	2
Heart failure, diastolic, acute	I5031	85	3
Heart failure, left	I501	85	2
Heart failure, systolic	I5020	85	2

COMORBID CONDITIONS

Comorbid Conditions	ICD-10	HCC	SOI
Heart failure, systolic, acute	I5021	85	3
Hematemesis	K920	-	2
Hemiplegia/hemiparesis	G8190	103	2
Hemiplegia/hemiparesis s/p CVA	I69359	103	2
Hemoptysis	R042	-	2
Hepatic encephalopathy, acute or subacute	K7200	-	**4**
Hepatic failure with coma	K7291	27	3
Hepatitis, chronic	*K739*	*29*	*-*
Hepatitis, viral	B199	-	-
Hepatorenal syndrome	K767	27	**4**
HIV disease/AIDS	B20	1	2
HIV positive	*Z21*	*1*	*-*
Hypercoagulable state, acquired	D68.69	48	2
Hypernatremia	E870	-	2
Hypertensive emergency/crisis	I161, I169	-	-
Hypertensive heart disease with heart failure	*I110*	*85*	*-*
Hyponatremia	E871	-	2
Ileus	K567	33	2
Immunocompromised/immunodeficient	D849	47	3
Immunodeficiency due to drugs	D84821	47	2
Impaction, rectal or intestinal	K5649	33	2
Intellectual disability, severe/profound	F72, F73	-	2
Intestinal obstruction	K56609	33	3
Jaundice	R17	-	2
Leukemia, in remission	C9591	10	-
Lung cancer	C3490	9	-
Lymphoma NOS	C8580	10	2
Malnutrition	E46	21	3
Malnutrition, mild	E441	21	3
Malnutrition, moderate	E440	21	3
Malnutrition, severe	E43	21	3

Comorbid Conditions	ICD-10	HCC	SOI
Metastatic cancer (secondary malignancies)	C770–C800	8	2
Morbid obesity	*E6601*	*22*	*-*
Multiple sclerosis	*G35*	*77*	*-*
Myelodysplastic syndrome	*D469*	*46*	*-*
Myocardial infarction, acute	I219	86	3
Myocardial injury, non-ischemic	I5A	-	2
Neurogenic bladder	G834	72	-
Neutropenia	*D709*	*47*	*2*
Obesity hypoventilation syndrome	E662	22	2
Opioid abuse with withdrawal	F1113	55	-
Opioid dependence	F1120	55	-
Opioid dependence, in remission	*F1121*	*55*	*-*
Pancreatic cyst, pseudocyst	K862, K863	-	3
Pancreatitis, acute	K8590	-	3
Pancreatitis, chronic	K861	34	-
Pancytopenia	D61818	47	3
Pancytopenia, due to chemo or drugs	D61810 D61811	47	3
Paraplegia	G8220	71	2
Parkinson's disease	*G20*	*78*	*-*
Peripheral vascular disease	*I739*	*108*	*-*
Peritoneal abscess	K651	33	**4**
Peritonitis	K659	33	3
Pneumonia	J189	-	2
Pneumonia, aspiration	J690	114	**4**
Pneumonia, other specified bacterial	J158	114	2
Pneumonia, due to chemical, fumes, vapors	J680	112	2
Pneumonia, aspiration post-procedural	J954	-	-
Pneumonia, VAP	J95851	114	**4**
Portal hypertension	K766	27	2

Comorbid Conditions	ICD-10	HCC	SOI
Pressure ulcer, Stage 3	L8993	158	2
Pressure ulcer, Stage 4	L8994	157	3
Pulmonary embolism, acute	I2699	107	4
Pulmonary embolism, chronic	I2782	107	2
Pulmonary heart disease	*I279*	*85*	*2*
Pulmonary hypertension	*I2720*	*85*	*2*
PSVT/PAT	I471	96	2
Quadriplegia	G8250	70	3
Quadriplegia, functional	R532	70	3
Resistance to antibiotics	Z1610-Z1639	-	-
Respiratory failure	J9690	84	4
Respiratory failure, acute	J9600	84	4
Respiratory failure, acute on chronic	J9620	84	4
Respiratory failure, postprocedural	J95821	84	4
Respiratory failure, chronic	J9610	84	3
Rhabdomyolysis	M6282	-	2
Rheumatoid arthritis	*M069*	*40*	-
Schatzki's ring, congenital	Q390	-	3
Schizophrenia	*F209*	*57*	-
Schizophrenia, simple, paranoid, residual	F2089	57	2
Sepsis	A419	2	3
Severe sepsis w/o septic shock	R6520	2	4
Severe sepsis with septic shock	R6521	2	4
Shock, unspecified	R579	84	3
Shock, cardiogenic (dc'd alive)	R570	84	4
Shock, hypovolemic (dc'd alive)	R571	2	4
Shock, septic (dc'd alive)	R6521	2	4

Comorbid Conditions	ICD-10	HCC	SOI
Shock, other (dc'd alive)	R578	2	4
Sick sinus syndrome	*I495*	*96*	*2*
Sickle cell disease	*D571*	*46*	*2*
SIRS, non-infectious	R6510	2	2
SIRS, non-infectious with organ dysfunction	R6511	2	**4**
Suicidal ideation	R45851	-	2
Supraventricular tachycardia (SVT)	I471	96	2
Thrombocytopenia	*D696*	*48*	*2*
Thrombophlebitis/phlebitis, deep vein	I80209	108	3
Thrombophlebitis/phlebitis, following infusion	T801XXA	-	2
Thrush, oral	B370	-	2
TIA (transient ischemic attack)	G459	-	2
Transplant status, bone marrow or stem cell	Z9481, Z9484	186	3
Transplant status, kidney	Z940	-	-
Transplant status, heart, lung, or liver	Z941, Z942 Z944	186	3 2
Ulcer, lower limb	L97909	161	2
Ulcerative colitis	K5190	35	-
Urinary tract infection (UTI)	N390	-	-
Ventricular fibrillation (dc'd alive)	I4901	84	3
Ventricular septal defect	Q210	-	-
Ventricular tachycardia	I472	96	2
Vertebral compression fracture, pathologic (non-traumatic)	M8008XA	169	2
Vertebral compression fracture, traumatic	S32009A	169	2
Weakness [hemiparesis] following CVA	I69359	103	2

The following is a listing of the more common diagnoses that are APR-DRG SOI-4 subclass. To achieve the highest score of 4 for severity of illness (SOI) and risk of mortality (ROM), e.g., for mortality reviews, typically two SOI-4 diagnoses, or one SOI-4 and two SOI-3 diagnoses, are necessary.

Diagnosis	ICD-10
Acute tubular necrosis	N170
Brain death	G9382
Brain injury, with LOC > 24 hours	S069X5A-S069X7A
Cardiac arrest (if POA)	I469
Cerebral edema	G936
Cerebral hemorrhage	I619
Cerebral infarction / CVA	I6350
Coma	R4020
Diabetes, hyperosmolar	E1100
Diabetes, with hypoglycemia & coma	E11641
Hepatic failure [encephalopathy], acute or subacute without coma	K7200
Hepatorenal syndrome	K767
Peritoneal abscess	K651
Pneumonia: aspiration or VAP	J690, J95851
Pulmonary embolism, acute	I2699
Respiratory failure	J9690
Severe sepsis without septic shock	R6520
Severe sepsis with septic shock	R6521
Shock: cardiogenic, hypovolemic, septic	R570, R571, R6521
SIRS, non-infectious with organ dysfunction	R6511

The table below includes the CMS-HCC Listing V24.0.

See **HCCs and Risk Adjustment** for more information.

HCC	HCC Description	Weight
1	HIV/AIDS	0.335
2	Septicemia, Sepsis, SIRS/Shock	0.352
6	Opportunistic Infections	0.424
8	Metastatic Cancer and Acute Leukemia	2.659
9	Lung and Other Severe Cancers	1.024
10	Lymphoma and Other Cancers	0.675
11	Colorectal, Bladder, and Other Cancers	0.307
12	Breast, Prostate, and Other Cancers and Tumors	0.150
17	Diabetes with Acute Complications	0.302
18	Diabetes with Chronic Complications	0.302
19	Diabetes without Complication	0.105
21	Protein-Calorie Malnutrition	0.455
22	Morbid Obesity	0.250
23	Other Significant Endocrine and Metabolic Disorders	0.194
27	End-Stage Liver Disease	0.882
28	Cirrhosis of Liver	0.363
29	Chronic Hepatitis	0.147
33	Intestinal Obstruction/Perforation	0.219
34	Chronic Pancreatitis	0.287
35	Inflammatory Bowel Disease	0.308
39	Bone/Joint/Muscle Infections/Necrosis	0.401
40	Rheumatoid Arthritis and Inflammatory Connective Tissue Disease	0.421
46	Severe Hematological Disorders	1.372

HCC	HCC Description	Weight
47	Disorders of Immunity	0.665
48	Coagulation Defects and Other Specified Hematological Disorders	0.192
51	Dementia with Complications	0.346
52	Dementia without Complications	0.346
54	Substance Use with Psychotic Complications	0.329
55	Substance Use Disorder, Moderate/Severe, or Substance Use with Complications	0.329
56	Substance Use Disorder, Mild, Except Alcohol and Cannabis	0.329
57	Schizophrenia	0.524
58	Reactive and Unspecified Psychosis	0.393
59	Major Depressive, Bipolar, and Paranoid Disorders	0.309
60	Personality Disorders	0.309
70	Quadriplegia	1.242
71	Paraplegia	1.068
72	Spinal Cord Disorders/Injuries	0.481
73	Amyotrophic Lateral Sclerosis and Other Motor Neuron Disease	0.999
74	Cerebral Palsy	0.339
75	Myasthenia Gravis/Myoneural Disorders and Guillain-Barre Syndrome/ Inflammatory and Toxic Neuropathy	0.472
76	Muscular Dystrophy	0.518
77	Multiple Sclerosis	0.423
78	Parkinson's and Huntington's Diseases	0.606
79	Seizure Disorders and Convulsions	0.220
80	Coma, Brain Compression/Anoxic Damage	0.486
82	Respirator Dependence/Tracheostomy Status	1.000
83	Respiratory Arrest	0.354

HCC	HCC Description	Weight
84	Cardio-Respiratory Failure and Shock	0.282
85	Congestive Heart Failure	0.331
86	Acute Myocardial Infarction	0.195
87	Unstable Angina and Other Acute Ischemic Heart Disease	0.195
88	Angina Pectoris	0.135
96	Specified Heart Arrhythmias	0.268
99	Intracranial Hemorrhage	0.230
100	Ischemic or Unspecified Stroke	0.230
103	Hemiplegia/Hemiparesis	0.437
104	Monoplegia, Other Paralytic Syndromes	0.331
106	Atherosclerosis of the Extremities with Ulceration or Gangrene	1.488
107	Vascular Disease with Complications	0.383
108	Vascular Disease	0.288
110	Cystic Fibrosis	0.510
111	Chronic Obstructive Pulmonary Disease	0.335
112	Fibrosis of Lung and Other Chronic Lung Disorders	0.219
114	Aspiration and Specified Bacterial Pneumonias	0.517
115	Pneumococcal Pneumonia, Empyema, Lung Abscess	0.130
122	Proliferative Diabetic Retinopathy and Vitreous Hemorrhage	0.222
124	Exudative Macular Degeneration	0.521
134	Dialysis Status	0.435
135	Acute Renal Failure	0.435
136	Chronic Kidney Disease, Stage 5	0.289
137	Chronic Kidney Disease, Severe (Stage 4)	0.289
138	Chronic Kidney Disease, Moderate (Stage 3)	0.069

HCC	HCC Description	Weight
157	Pressure Ulcer of Skin with Necrosis Through to Muscle, Tendon, or Bone	2.028
158	Pressure Ulcer of Skin with Full Thickness Skin Loss	1.069
159	Pressure Ulcer of Skin with Partial Thickness Skin Loss	0.656
161	Chronic Ulcer of Skin, Except Pressure	0.515
162	Severe Skin Burn or Condition	0.224
166	Severe Head Injury	0.486
167	Major Head Injury	0.077
169	Vertebral Fractures without Spinal Cord Injury	0.476
170	Hip Fracture/Dislocation	0.350
173	Traumatic Amputations and Complications	0.208
176	Complications of Specified Implanted Device or Graft	0.582
186	Major Organ Transplant or Replacement Status	0.832
188	Artificial Openings for Feeding or Elimination	0.534
189	Amputation Status, Lower Limb/Amputation Complications	0.519

Weights for V24.0 Community, Non-Dual, Age-eligible Medicare.

Height	Body weight (in pounds)													
4'10"	91	96	100	105	110	115	119	124	129	134	138	143	167	191
4'11"	94	99	104	109	114	119	124	128	133	138	143	148	173	198
5'0"	97	102	107	112	118	123	128	133	138	143	148	153	179	204
5'1"	100	106	111	116	122	127	132	137	143	148	153	158	185	211
5'2"	104	109	115	120	126	131	136	142	147	153	158	164	191	218
5'3"	107	113	118	124	130	135	141	146	152	158	163	169	197	225
5'4"	110	116	122	128	134	140	145	151	157	163	169	174	204	232
5'5"	114	120	126	132	138	144	150	156	162	168	174	180	210	240
5'6"	118	124	130	136	142	148	155	161	167	173	179	186	216	247
5'7"	121	127	134	140	146	153	159	166	172	178	185	191	223	255
5'8"	125	131	138	144	151	158	164	171	177	184	190	197	230	262
5'9"	128	135	142	149	155	162	169	176	182	189	196	203	236	270
5'10"	132	139	146	153	160	167	174	181	188	195	202	209	243	278
5'11"	136	143	150	157	165	172	179	186	193	200	208	215	250	286
6'0"	140	147	154	162	169	177	184	191	199	206	213	221	258	294
6'1"	144	151	159	166	174	182	189	197	204	212	219	227	265	302
6'2"	148	155	163	171	179	186	194	202	210	218	225	233	272	311
6'3"	152	160	168	176	184	192	200	208	216	224	232	240	279	319
6'4"	156	164	172	180	189	197	205	213	221	230	238	246	287	328
BMI	**19**	**20**	**21**	**22**	**23**	**24**	**25**	**26**	**27**	**28**	**29**	**30**	**35**	**40**
	NORMAL						OVERWEIGHT					OBESE		

OVERVIEW

This section lists particular DRGs that could potentially be reassigned to an alternative DRG. The list is not all-inclusive; a DRG not included in this section may still have opportunities to improve the DRG assignment.

For all medical DRGs, always LOOK FOR an **alternative principal diagnosis** based on the definition of the principal diagnosis or sequencing guidelines per coding rules.

Refer to the *Comorbid Conditions* section for commonly associated or missed comorbidities.

For each DRG, the following is included:

- Alternative DRGs
- Alternate or more specific principal diagnoses
- Commonly associated CCs or MCCs
- Other or more specific surgical or non-operating room procedures
- Reference to the specific *Key Reference* topic for the clinical indicators and further guidance.

DRG 60   **Multiple Sclerosis w/o CC/MCC**

LOOK FOR pain or loss of vision due to optic neuritis (H46.9) as a secondary diagnosis that is often associated with multiple sclerosis.

DRG 64   **Cerebral Hemorrhage/Infarction w MCC**
DRG 65   **Cerebral Hemorrhage/Infarction w CC or TPA in 24 hrs**
DRG 66   **Cerebral Hemorrhage/Infarction w/o CC/MCC**

PRINCIPAL DIAGNOSIS

LOOK FOR evidence of trauma causing intracranial hemorrhage and loss of consciousness for alternative DRGs 85-87 or 82-84, Traumatic Stupor & Coma. Subdural hematoma usually means trauma, and commonly occurs in the elderly and alcoholics.

MCC

LOOK FOR cerebral edema (G93.6), brain compression (G93.5), or coma (R40.20). See *Cerebral Edema/Compression* or *Coma.*

CC

LOOK FOR right or left-sided weakness (coded as hemiparesis), hemiparesis or hemiplegia due to CVA (I69.959). Residual from old stroke or caused by a new acute CVA (even if resolved at the time of hospital discharge) can be coded.

LOOK FOR tPA. If patient received tPA (tissue plasminogen activator) at prior facility within last 24 hours, add code Z92.82 for DRG 65.

PROCEDURE

If TPA infusion (3E03317), DRG 61-63, Ischemic stroke, precerebral occlusion or TIA with thrombolytic agent, is assigned.

DRG 69   Transient Ischemic Attack

PRINCIPAL DIAGNOSIS

LOOK FOR persistent neurologic deficit > 24 hours (despite negative imaging study), or positive imaging study (MRI/CT) which is a CVA for DRGs 64-66, Cerebral infarction.

LOOK FOR TIA caused by cerebral or precerebral stenosis, occlusion and cerebral embolism which are assigned to DRGs 67-68, Nonspecific CVA & precerebral occlusion w/o infarct, having greater severity than TIA.

LOOK FOR another diagnosis that is more specific than TIA such as "transient global ischemia" (G45.4) which is assigned to DRGs 70–72, Nonspecific cerebrovascular disorders.

PROCEDURE

LOOK FOR for TPA infusion (3E03317). TIA or precerebral occlusion with TPA infusion are assigned to DRGs 61-63, Ischemic stroke, precerebral occlusion or TIA with thrombolytic agent.

DRG 70-72   Nonspecific Cerebrovascular Disorders

PRINCIPAL DIAGNOSIS

Encephalopathy is the principal diagnosis mostly commonly assigned to these DRGs 70-72.

LOOK FOR hepatic encephalopathy, hepatic failure, hepatitis, or other hepatic disorder as reason for admission for DRG 441-443, Disorders of liver except malig, cirr, alc hepatitis, or DRG 432-434, Cirrhosis & alcoholic hepatitis. Hepatic encephalopathy or failure are potentially life-threatening conditions. Note that patients are not typically admitted for liver cirrhosis itself (in the absence of bleeding varices) since this is a chronic condition. See ***Hepatic Encephalopathy & Failure***.

<u>LOOK FOR</u> poisoning as the cause of the encephalopathy. Poisoning is an adverse reaction to a medication taken improperly. If poisoning, the poisoning code is sequenced first with toxic encephalopathy (if specified) code G92.9 as MCC for DRG 917, Poisoning & toxic effects of drugs w MCC.

<u>LOOK FOR</u> toxic encephalopathy due to alcohol intoxication, or due to the effects of medications and toxins for DRG 917 (Poisoning & toxic effects of drugs w MCC). Alcohol intoxication is coded as T51.0X1A with G92.9 (toxic encephalopathy) as secondary diagnosis. If due to a poisoning or toxin, the poisoning code (T36-T50) or toxic effect code (T51-T65) is sequenced first followed by G92.9. See *Adverse Reactions to Drugs & Toxins.*

<u>LOOK FOR</u> diabetic hypoglycemia as cause of encephalopathy for DRG 637, Diabetes w MCC. Diabetic hypoglycemia is coded to E11.649 and G93.41 (if specified as metabolic encephalopathy). Although "Encephalopathy, hypoglycemic" is indexed to E16.2, hypoglycemia unspecified, it is not assigned with diabetes (see Excludes 1 note).

UTI (N39.0) is commonly associated with encephalopathy and is not usually the principal reason for admission.

DRG 100   **Seizures w MCC**
DRG 101   **Seizures w/o MCC**

PRINCIPAL DIAGNOSIS
Seizures may be either primary (seizure disorder) or a secondary symptom or manifestation of an underlying disease.

<u>LOOK FOR</u> underlying cause of seizures, e.g., brain tumor (primary or metastatic) as alternate principal diagnosis for DRGs 54-55, Nervous system neoplasms.

<u>LOOK FOR</u> cerebral infarction or precerebral occlusion as underlying cause of seizure for DRGs 64-66, Cerebral infarction, or DRGs 67-68, Nonspecific CVA & precerebral occlusion w/o infarct.

<u>LOOK FOR</u> an infectious cause of the seizures, such as meningitis, HIV, viral encephalitis, etc.

DRG 149   Dysequilibrium

PRINCIPAL DIAGNOSIS

<u>LOOK FOR</u> the cause of dysequilibrium such as:

- Anemia or blood loss anemia as cause of dizziness for DRG 811-812 (Anemia). Check for occult stool blood or if Hct < 30/Hgb < 10, transfusion.

- Precerebral/cerebral occlusion or stenosis as cause of dysequilibrium/TIA for DRG 67-68, Precerebral occlusions.

- TIA (or CVA) as cause of symptoms for DRG 69, TIA. Cerebellar ischemia (vertebro-basilar arteries) or unilateral weakness causing dysequilibrium < 24 hours duration.

- Syncope/presyncope or orthostatic hypotension as alternate principal diagnosis for DRG 312, Syncope. Review the record for evidence suggesting syncope, near-syncope or vaso-vagal hypotension.

- Dehydration, hypovolemia, other electrolyte imbalance for DRGs 640-641, Electrolyte disorders, are common causes of dizziness and vertigo. Verify lab values (BUN, Na, K); look for poor skin turgor, IV fluids.

- Diabetes or uncontrolled diabetes as reason for admission for DRGs 637-639, Diabetes. Glucose > 400, ketosis, hyperosmolar, insulin or oral meds adjustment, endocrine consult.

| DRG 150 | **Epistaxis w MCC** |
| DRG 151 | **Epistaxis w/o MCC** |

PRINCIPAL DIAGNOSIS

Verify reason for admission and principal diagnosis. Typically, patients are not admitted for uncomplicated epistaxis (nose bleed) and are more appropriately placed in observation.

LOOK FOR underlying cause such as thrombocytopenia or coagulopathy (hereditary, acquired or consequence of medical therapy) for DRG 813. A common cause of epistasis is the side-effect of over-anticoagulation with Coumadin, in which case epistaxis is sequenced first. Occasionally Coumadin is taken incorrectly (poisoning): the poisoning code would be sequenced first (DRGs 917-918). See *Coagulation Disorders.*

| DRG 152 | **Otitis Media & URI w MCC** |
| DRG 153 | **Otitis Media & URI w/o MCC** |

PRINCIPAL DIAGNOSIS

LOOK FOR alternative reason for admission or further specificity of principal diagnosis. Patients are not typically admitted for otitis media, upper respiratory infection, acute sinusitis, laryngitis, uncomplicated influenza.

LOOK FOR complications of influenza as reason for admission or with pneumonia. Influenza is assigned to DRGs 193-195, Simple pneumonia.

DRG 177-179 **Respiratory Infections**

PRINCIPAL DIAGNOSIS

LOOK FOR sepsis criteria for DRG 871, Septicemia or severe sepsis. Sepsis is usually sequenced first if present on admission. Pneumonia is MCC when sepsis is principal diagnosis.

MCC

LOOK FOR diagnostic criteria for respiratory failure.

PROCEDURE

LOOK FOR intubation and ventilation for DRGs 207-208, Respiratory system diagnosis with ventilator support.

DRG 180-182 **Respiratory Neoplasms**

PRINCIPAL DIAGNOSIS

LOOK FOR "complex" pneumonia, HCAP, "post-obstructive" pneumonia as reason for admission for DRGs 177-179, Respiratory infections. Unspecified pneumonia may be documented but antibiotics for gram-negative and/or staph given (such as Zosyn and vancomycin). See *Pneumonia*.

CC

LOOK FOR malignant pleural effusion; symptoms, complication, evaluation or treatment.

PROCEDURE

LOOK FOR transbronchial biopsy performed with bronchoscopy (ex. 0BBJ8ZX) for DRGs 166-168, Other resp system O.R. procedures. Review procedure and pathology report. See *Transbronchial Biopsy*.

DRG 189   Pulmonary Edema & Respiratory Failure

PRINCIPAL DIAGNOSIS

LOOK FOR acute heart failure as co-equal principal diagnosis for DRG 291, Heart failure & shock w MCC. Although acute respiratory failure may be due to acute heart failure, sequencing depends on the circumstances and focus of the admission. Acute respiratory failure is typically the focus of the admission when patient is on a ventilator for DRG 207-208, Respiratory system diagnosis with ventilator support.

PROCEDURE

LOOK FOR intubation, mechanical ventilation for DRG 207-208, Respiratory system diagnosis with ventilator support.

DRG 190-192 **COPD**

PRINCIPAL DIAGNOSIS

LOOK FOR pneumonia or evidence of pneumonia for 193-195, Simple pneumonia, or 177-179, Respiratory infection. If COPD and pneumonia are co-equal, sequencing depends upon the circumstances of admission. Treatment of simple pneumonia and COPD likely to be the same: antibiotics, O2, IV steroids, other respiratory care. See *Pneumonia*.

LOOK FOR diagnostic criteria for acute respiratory failure for DRG 189, Pulmonary edema & respiratory failure, or as an MCC. Sequencing depends on circumstances and focus of admission.

LOOK FOR respiratory neoplasm as interrelated principal diagnosis for DRG 180-182, Respiratory neoplasms. Respiratory problems could be due to progression of respiratory malignancy. If diagnosed or treated on current admission, sequence neoplasm as principal diagnosis.

MCC

LOOK FOR acute respiratory failure commonly occurs with acute exacerbation of COPD and would typically be expected in status asthmaticus.

CC

LOOK FOR indicators of chronic respiratory failure, e.g., "severe COPD on home O2." See ***Respiratory Failure–Chronic & Acute on Chronic.***

PROCEDURE

LOOK FOR transbronchial biopsy performed for DRGs 166-168, Other respiratory system OR procedures. See ***Transbronchial Biopsy.***

LOOK FOR intubation and mechanical ventilation for DRGs 207-208, Respiratory system diagnosis with ventilatory support.

DRG 193-195 **Simple Pneumonia**

PRINCIPAL DIAGNOSIS

LOOK FOR clinical indicators of gram-negative, staph, or aspiration pneumonia for DRGs 177-179, Respiratory infections. HCAP, CAP, or unspecified pneumonia may be documented but antibiotics for gram-negative and/or staph given (such as Zosyn and vancomycin), so a query for probable/suspected organism or aspiration is necessary.

LOOK FOR sepsis criteria for DRG 871, Septicemia or severe sepsis. Sepsis is usually sequenced first if present on admission. Pneumonia is MCC when sepsis is principal diagnosis.

LOOK FOR acute exacerbation of COPD (AECOPD) for DRG 190, COPD. If pneumonia is co-equal with COPD and no other MCC, sequence AECOPD as principal diagnosis and pneumonia as secondary; if another MCC, sequence pneumonia as principal diagnosis. Treatment of pneumonia and COPD is likely to be the same: antibiotics, O2 therapy, IV steroids, other respiratory care modalities. See ***Asthma/Bronchitis/COPD.***

LOOK FOR diagnostic criteria for **acute respiratory failure** for DRG 189, Pulmonary edema & respiratory failure, or as an MCC. Sequencing depends on the circumstances and focus of admission.

LOOK FOR diagnostic criteria for **chronic respiratory failure**. See *Respiratory Failure–Chronic & Acute on Chronic.*

LOOK FOR **antibiotic resistance** (K16.10-K16.39) in the culture results or progress notes.

DRG 202   **Bronchitis & Asthma w CC/MCC**
DRG 203   **Bronchitis & Asthma w/o CC/MCC**

PRINCIPAL DIAGNOSIS
LOOK FOR acute bronchitis with COPD (J44.0) or bronchiectasis (J47.0) or asthma with COPD (J44.9), i.e., history of COPD, COPD on chest x-ray, history of chronic or recurrent bronchitis for DRGs 190-192, COPD.

LOOK FOR evidence of pneumonia for DRGs 193-195, Simple pneumonia & pleurisy. See *Pneumonia.*

LOOK FOR more specific condition that is causing the symptoms or "status asthmaticus" which often indicates acute respiratory failure.

DRG 204   **Respiratory Signs & Symptoms**

PRINCIPAL DIAGNOSIS
Verify that the most specific diagnosis is used as principal diagnosis considering all alternative medical DRGs. Selection of a symptom code is primarily the reason for assignment to this DRG, such as dyspnea, shortness of breath, acute respiratory distress, hemoptysis, apnea, etc. LOOK FOR a cause or potential cause of the symptom.

DRG 207   **Resp System Diagnoses w Vent 96+ hrs**
DRG 208   **Resp System Diagnoses w Vent <96 hrs**

PRINCIPAL DIAGNOSIS
Verify documentation adequately supports a respiratory diagnosis as
principal diagnosis to ensure appropriate assignment to these DRGs.

PROCEDURE
Carefully calculate duration of ventilation (start/end time) of
ventilation if > 3 days to verify 96 hour benchmark. See *Mechanical
Ventilation*.

DRG 247   **Perc CV Proc w Drug Eluting Stent w/o MCC**
DRG 249   **Perc CV Proc w Non-Drug Eluting Stent w/o MCC**

PRINCIPAL DIAGNOSIS
Verify reason for admission. Patients should be admitted emergently
with an acute condition, e.g., unstable angina, acute MI, heart failure.
High risk for medical necessity denial if stent not done urgently. If
admitted following outpatient surgery, the complication should be the
principal diagnosis.

MCC
LOOK FOR acute MI, reperfusion injury, or other complications following
PCI/stent insertion as MCCs occurring during admission.

PROCEDURE
Review the content of the operative report carefully to determine the
number of arteries and stents involved: 4 or more arteries or stents is
equivalent to an MCC for DRGs 246 or 248, Perc CV proc w stent w
MCC or 4+ arteries/stents.

DRG 252-254 **Other Vascular Procedures**

PRINCIPAL DIAGNOSIS

Verify reason for admission, such as postop complication as reason for admission from ambulatory surgery or additional procedures. When not urgent condition, these procedures are often performed on outpatient basis. LOOK FOR postop ATN or AKI as reason for inpatient admission from ambulatory surgery.

MCC OR CC

LOOK FOR clinical indicators for AKI and ATN. Acute renal failure following IV contrast occurs commonly which is due to ATN.

DRG 255-257 **Upper Limb & Toe Amputation for Circ Syst Disorders**

PRINCIPAL DIAGNOSIS

LOOK FOR a diabetic complication as principal diagnosis when toe amputation performed, e.g., skin ulcer with DM (E11.622), osteomyelitis with DM (E11.69), for DRGs 616-618, Amputation of lower limb for endocrine, nutrit, & metabolic dis.

DRG 280-282 **Acute Myocardial Infarction**

MCC

LOOK FOR evidence of acute systolic/diastolic heart failure which is often associated with acute MI. Dyspnea, hypoxia, rales, wheezing, "volume overload," left ventricular dysfunction. This can be sequenced as either principal or secondary diagnosis for MCC and DRG 280 is assigned. See **Heart Failure.**

CC

LOOK FOR cardiac arrhythmia following MI, such as Vtach, SVT, PAT, Atrial flutter. Often in telemetry strips, nursing notes, progress notes.

Vtach = 3 or more consecutive ventricular beats at a rate > 120; almost always significant and "monitored." See *Cardiac Dysrhythmia*.

LOOK FOR chronic systolic/diastolic heart failure.

LOOK FOR pericarditis following acute MI — Dressler's Syndrome. Clinical signs include pleuritic chest pain, pericardial "friction rub," fever and/or elevated sed rate (ESR).

PROCEDURE

LOOK FOR insertion of coronary stent (drug-eluting or non-drug eluting) for DRGs 247 or 249, Perc CV proc w drug-eluting/non-drug eluting stent. Review the content of the operative report carefully to determine the number of arteries or stents involved: 4 or more arteries or stents is equivalent to an MCC and assigned to DRG 246 or 248, Perc CV proc w MCC or 4+ arteries or stents.

DRG 291-293 **Heart Failure**

PRINCIPAL DIAGNOSIS

LOOK FOR documentation of hypertension and CKD (I13.0) in patients admitted principally for acute heart failure. Code I13.0 becomes principal diagnosis and the acute heart failure becomes a secondary diagnosis for DRG 291, Heart failure with MCC. See *Heart Failure.*

LOOK FOR indicators of acute MI in addition to or associated with heart failure. Whether acute MI is assigned as secondary or principal diagnosis, DRG 280, Acute myocardial infarction, dc'd alive, is assigned. See *Myocardial Injury, Ischemia, Infarction*.

LOOK FOR acute respiratory failure as principal diagnosis when patient is intubated and on ventilator for DRGs 207-208, Respiratory system diagnosis with vent support. Although respiratory failure may be due to acute heart failure, sequencing depends on the circumstances and focus of the admission. Acute respiratory failure is typically the focus of the admission when patient is on a ventilator.

MCC OR **CC**

LOOK FOR diagnostic criteria for acute or chronic respiratory failure.

DRG 296-298 **Cardiac Arrest, Unexplained**

PRINCIPAL DIAGNOSIS

Cardiac arrest is unlikely to be principal diagnosis when the patient is resuscitated and survives to be admitted. If the cause is known, such as myocardial infarction, the cause would be sequenced first, for DRG 280, Acute MI, dc alive w MCC. If the cause, such as ventricular fibrillation, was corrected prior to admission, cardiac arrest would not typically be the focus of the admission pursuant to OCG II.B and C (circumstances of admission, therapy provided).

Most often the reason for admission is a consequence of the cardiac arrest and the most likely principal diagnosis. In fact, the cardiac arrest often resolves prior to admission. For example, a patient in cardiac arrest resuscitated in the emergency room and admitted with respiratory failure (on a ventilator or not) is assigned to DRG 189 (Pulmonary edema & respiratory failure) or DRGs 207-208, Resp system diagnosis with ventilator support, if placed on a ventilator. See ***Cardiac Arrest.***

DRG 308-310 **Cardiac Arrhythmia & Conduction Disorders**

PRINCIPAL DIAGNOSIS

LOOK FOR a co-equal principal diagnosis such as heart failure, etc.

LOOK FOR cardiac arrhythmia due to malfunction of cardiac device. For example, ventricular tachycardia caused by malfunction of defibrillator (didn't fire) would be assigned code T82.118A, complication of cardiac electronic device and assigned to DRGs 314-316, Other circulatory system diagnoses.

MCC
LOOK FOR type 2 MI (I21.A1) with elevated troponins for DRG 282, Acute MI.

DRG 311   **Angina Pectoris**

PRINCIPAL DIAGNOSIS
LOOK FOR CAD. A cause and effect relationship may be assumed when a patient has both CAD and angina and a combination code is assigned (I25.119) for DRGs 302-303, Atherosclerosis.

Acute coronary syndrome (ACS) is coded as unstable angina, but if with elevated troponins, LOOK FOR an MI (NSTEMI) for DRGs 280-282. See *Myocardial Injury, Ischemia, Infarction.*

DRG 312   **Syncope & Collapse**

PRINCIPAL DIAGNOSIS
Syncope is a symptom and defined as transient loss of consciousness without subsequent sequelae. Most common cause (if not due to orthostatic hypotension) is cardiac arrhythmia, which may be difficult to diagnose without prolonged cardiac event monitoring, particularly when no cause is identified by the initial work-up. In this case, a query is usually warranted for possible or suspected arrhythmia as the likely cause.

LOOK FOR
- Significant **tachycardia, bradycardia or heart block** (2nd or 3rd degree) for DRGs 308-310, Cardiac arrhythmia. These conditions may cause hypotension with resulting syncope. First degree and 2nd degree heart block (Mobitz I) usually have no symptoms and do not cause syncope, although they may be harbingers of a higher degree of heart block especially if any type of bundle branch block is also present.

- **Acute blood loss anemia** caused by acute hemorrhage for DRGs 811-812, Anemia. Chronic anemia usually develops gradually and is well tolerated until it becomes severe (H/H < 8/24). Evaluation of chronic GI blood loss in stable patients may be conducted on an outpatient basis.
- **Electrolyte imbalance** or dehydration for DRGs 640-641, Electrolyte disorders. If elevated creatinine, may be acute kidney injury. Patients with simple dehydration and/or minor electrolyte abnormalities are likely candidates for observation status.
- **Hypoglycemia** for DRGs 637-639, Diabetes. Low blood sugar does not usually cause unconsciousness/syncope unless < 40 and is almost always due to insulin or oral diabetic medication (adverse effect or poisoning). Rx: Oral or parenteral glucose administration, glucagon, modification of diabetic medications. Patients with uncomplicated hypoglycemia are likely candidates for observation. If due to long-acting oral meds inpatient likely needed.
- **Stenosis of vertebrobasilar** (VB) or rarely bilateral carotid arteries for DRGs 67-68, Precerebral occlusions w/o infarct. Thrombosis/embolism is not a likely cause of syncope. The usual warning sign of VB stenosis is syncope. VB syndrome or insufficiency is classified as TIA, so an opportunity to query for stenosis as underlying cause.
- **Autonomic neuropathy** due to any condition may cause syncope, although diabetes is a very common cause. Autonomic neuropathy or diabetic neuropathy specified as cause of syncope are assigned to DRGs 73-74, Cranial & peripheral nerve disorders.

DRG 313   Chest Pain

PRINCIPAL DIAGNOSIS
Inpatient admission is usually not necessary for non-specific chest pain or for simple "rule-out MI". Such cases have a high risk for denial.

LOOK FOR possible cause of the chest pain for other medical DRGs.

DRG 341-343 Appendectomy w/o Complicated PDX

PRINCIPAL DIAGNOSIS

LOOK FOR "**peritonitis**" with "**abscess**" in pre- or postop documentation including CT reports and in operative note. Reference to "exudate," "purulence," "serositis," or similar terms, especially when small bowel involved for DRGs 338-340, Appendectomy with complicated PDX.

Complicated PDX with acute appendicitis: K35.21 (with generalized pertonitis and abscess), K35.32 (with perforation and localized peritonitis), or malignancy of appendix (C18.1 or C7A020).

LOOK FOR clinical criteria for **sepsis** for DRGs 853-854, Infectious & parasitic disease w O.R. procedure. Surgeons do not customarily consider healthy, "non-toxic" patients with simple, uncomplicated appendicitis to have sepsis even when fever, tachycardia, and leukocytosis may be present, since these are clinically intrinsic to the diagnosis. The same may not be true for elderly or chronically ill individuals or those with perforation/abscess where sepsis may occur. A patient with multiple sepsis indicators and/or toxic-appearing may have sepsis.

PROCEDURE

LOOK FOR lysis of adhesions (ex. 0DNW4ZZ) for DRGs 335-337, Peritoneal adhesiolysis. Must be extensive or dense requiring significant surgical effort such as resection, enterotomy, substantial "take-down," bowel obstruction, or otherwise altering the procedure. Do not code based solely on mention of adhesions or simple lysis in the operative report.

DRG 344-346 Minor Small & Large Bowel Procedures

PROCEDURE

Although the root operation for "takedown, stoma" is "reposition," look also for an "**excision**" of the bowel, for DRGs 329-331, Major small & large bowel procedures. For example, in ileostomy closure both ends of the intestines are typically excised (0DBB0ZZ) before the anastomosis. See *Coding Clinic 2016 Q3 p. 3.*

DRG 350-352 Ing & Femoral Hernia Procedures

PRINCIPAL DIAGNOSIS

LOOK FOR a **complication** or other condition as reason for admission following ambulatory surgery, such as cardiac arrhythmia, atelectasis, etc. In these cases, the surgical diagnosis would be a secondary diagnosis and the surgical procedure also coded for DRGs 987-989, Non-extensive O.R. procedure unrelated to PDX.

PROCEDURE

LOOK FOR other type of hernia repaired for DRGs 353-355, Hernia procedures *except* ing & femoral. If not inguinal or femoral hernia repair, principal diagnosis code and procedure code will change.

LOOK FOR lysis of adhesions (ex. 0DNW4ZZ) for DRGs 335-337, Peritoneal adhesiolysis. Must be extensive or dense requiring significant surgical effort such as resection, enterotomy, substantial "take-down," bowel obstruction, or otherwise altering the procedure. Do not code based solely on mention of adhesions or simple lysis in the operative report.

DRG 353-355 Hernia Proc except Inguinal & Femoral

PRINCIPAL DIAGNOSIS

LOOK FOR **failed mesh graft** (T85.698A) as principal diagnosis or repeat incisional or ventral hernia repair for failed mesh graft for DRGs 907-909, Other O.R. procedures for injuries.

PROCEDURE

LOOK FOR **manipulation** of intestine (reposition colon) for DRGs 344-346, Minor small & large bowel procedures. Hernia repairs may include reduction of the bowel. A torsed, twisted, or kinked bowel may require a manipulation or manual correction.

LOOK FOR lysis of adhesions for DRGs 335-337, Peritoneal adhesiolysis. Must be extensive or dense requiring significant surgical effort such as resection, enterotomy, substantial "take-down," bowel obstruction, or otherwise altering the procedure. Do not code based solely on mention of adhesions or simple lysis in the operative report.

DRG 377-379 **GI Hemorrhage**

PRINCIPAL DIAGNOSIS

LOOK FOR evidence of **esophagitis** (K20.91) or **GERD with esophagitis** (K21.01) on endoscopy report for DRGs 368-370, Major esophageal disorders. The "with" rule presumes a causal relationship between these diagnoses and GI bleeding (unless another cause of GI bleeding is specified).

LOOK FOR **esophageal varices** which are almost always due to liver cirrhosis (alcoholic or non-alcoholic) with associated portal hypertension for DRG 432, Cirrhosis & alcoholic hepatitis w MCC. For patients with esophageal varices in or due to cirrhosis or certain other liver diseases or portal hypertension, *code first* the underlying disease, e.g., liver cirrhosis.

LOOK FOR evidence of **malignancy** as cause of GI bleed for DRGs 374-376, Digestive malignancy. Underlying malignancy must be treated, evaluated or undergoing workup to be sequenced as principal diagnosis. See *Neoplasms*.

LOOK FOR **acute blood loss anemia** almost always associated with GI hemorrhage. See *Acute Blood Loss Anemia*.

| DRG 383 | **Uncomplicated Peptic Ulcer w MCC** |
| DRG 384 | **Uncomplicated Peptic Ulcer w/o MCC** |

PRINCIPAL DIAGNOSIS

LOOK FOR **esophageal ulcer** or **erosions** (K22.10) or **Barrett's esophagus** (K22.70) on UGI or endoscopy for DRGs 380-382, Complicated peptic ulcer.

DRG 385-387 **Inflammatory Bowel Disease**

PRINCIPAL DIAGNOSIS

LOOK FOR enteritis/colitis due to Clostridium difficile (A04.72), Campylobacter (A04.5), E. coli (A04.4), or bacterial (A04.9) for DRGs 371-373, Major GI disorders & peritoneal infections. These are infections of the bowel that may cause severe diarrhea (often bloody), dehydration, and/or electrolyte imbalance. May be fatal especially in the elderly. See *Clostridium Difficile Infection*.

E. coli is a common form of travelers' diarrhea. Campylobacter is similar to C. diff. Bacterial colitis is also similar to the above but less specific. Sepsis not unusual with these infections.

| DRG 391 | **Esophagitis, Gastroenteritis & Digestive Dis w MCC** |
| DRG 392 | **Esophagitis, Gastroenteritis & Digestive Dis w/o MCC** |

PRINCIPAL DIAGNOSIS

LOOK FOR diabetic **gastroparesis** (E11.43) for DRGs 73-74, Cranial & peripheral nerve disorders. Very common manifestation of diabetes: usually vomiting without diarrhea; dilated stomach/abdominal pressure; frequently spontaneous without precipitating event, tends to be recurrent and caused by autonomic neuropathy. Often overlooked or confused with gastritis, peptic disease, other GI disorders. Rx: Reglan (metoclopramide) is the best treatment, and very specific for gastroparesis.

LOOK FOR **radiation** or **toxic gastroenteritis/colitis** (K52.0, K52.1) or ischemic colitis (K55.9) for DRGs 393-395, Other digestive system diagnoses. Symptoms of radiation/toxic gastritis are diarrhea, pain, bleeding, obstruction secondary to radiation therapy or toxin. Ischemic colitis = ischemic changes of mucosa of colon or small bowel due to loss of blood supply.

LOOK FOR evidence of **ileus** or bowel obstruction on imaging for DRGs 388-390, GI obstruction. Constipation, obstipation. RX: NPO, IVF, NG tube.

LOOK FOR **C. diff enteritis/colitis** or other bacterial colitis for DRGs 371-373, Major GI disorders & peritoneal infections. Includes Clostridium difficile (A04.72), Campylobacter (A04.5), E. coli (A04.4), or bacterial (A04.9) enteritis. See *Clostridium Difficile Infection.*

LOOK FOR **esophageal ulcer** or **erosions** (K22.10) for DRGs 380-382, Complicated peptic ulcer. Endoscopy or UGI indicates esophageal ulcer or erosions, or diagnosis of ulcer with obstruction.

LOOK FOR villous **adenomas** (D37.9) for DRGs 374-376, Digestive malignancy. These tumors secrete large amounts of mucous causing abdominal pain and diarrhea.

LOOK FOR gastric, peptic, duodenal **ulcer** as cause of gastroenteritis, abdominal pain, and/or vomiting for DRGs 383-384, Uncomplicated peptic ulcer. Endoscopy or x-ray may indicate ulcer or stress ulcer. RX: Tagamet, Pepcid, Carafate.

LOOK FOR **GI bleeding** or melena for DRGs 377-379, G.I. hemorrhage, or esophagitis "with" bleeding for DRGs 368-370, Major Esophageal Disorders. Drop in H/H, anemia, or blood in stool may indicate evidence of GI bleeding.

LOOK FOR **Crohn's disease** (regional enteritis) or **ulcerative colitis** for DRGs 385-387, Inflammatory bowel disease. Colicky pain, bowel obstruction (partial or complete); diarrhea, often bloody. RX: antibiotics, steroids, sulfa-derivatives, anti-metabolites, TNF inhibitors.

DRG 393-395 **Other Digestive System Diagnoses**

Verify principal diagnosis. Be sure the principal diagnosis accurately reflects the reason for admission and acuity. Inpatient admission is not usually required for many of the conditions that are assigned to this DRG, such as colon polyps, hernia, hemorrhoids, anal abscess, unless there is GI bleeding or surgery performed.

DRG 417-419 **Lap Cholecystectomy w/o C.D.E.**

PRINCIPAL DIAGNOSIS

LOOK FOR complication or other condition following ambulatory surgery as reason for admission (and principal diagnosis), such as cardiac arrhythmia. In these cases, the surgical diagnosis would be listed as a secondary diagnosis and the surgical procedure also coded and appropriately assigned to DRG 987-989, Non-extensive O.R. procedure unrelated to principal diagnosis.

PROCEDURE

LOOK FOR lap cholecystectomy converted to an **open** cholecystectomy for DRGs 414-416 or 411-413, Cholecystectomy w or w/o C.D.E. Check op note for common bile duct exploration (ex. 0FJB4ZZ).

DRG 432-434 **Cirrhosis & Alcoholic Hepatitis**

PRINCIPAL DIAGNOSIS

LOOK FOR **hepatic encephalopathy** or failure as reason for admission for DRG 441-443, Disorders of liver except malig, cirr, alc hepa. In the absence of bleeding varices, patients are not typically admitted for

liver cirrhosis itself since this is a chronic condition. Hepatic encephalopathy, failure or coma are potentially life-threatening conditions.

| DRG 459 | **Spinal Fusion exc Cervical w MCC** |
| DRG 460 | **Spinal Fusion exc Cervical w/o MCC** |

PRINCIPAL DIAGNOSIS

<u>LOOK FOR</u> an alternate principal diagnosis for DRGs 456-458, Spinal
fusion w spinal curv/malig/infection or ext fusion, such as scoliosis
(M41.9) or chronic osteomyelitis (M46.20), or kyphosis (M40.209),
or curvature of spine (M43.9) due to or associated with another
condition. The underlying disease that caused the kyphosis, such as
osteoporosis, would be coded first.

| DRG 468 | **Revision of Hip or Knee Replacement w/o CC/MCC** |

Acute blood loss anemia. Significant blood loss anemia following
major orthopedic surgery is common. Check for drop in Hgb/Hct
below normal or preop baseline. See *Acute Blood Loss Anemia*.

| DRG 469 | **Major Joint Replacement or LE Reatt w MCC** |
| DRG 470 | **Major Joint Replacement or LE Reatt w/o MCC** |

PROCEDURE

Bilateral joint replacements require two codes (right and left) for
DRGs 461-462, Bilateral or multiple major joint procedures of lower
extremity.

DRG 480-482 **Hip & Femur Proc Exc Major Joint**

PRINCIPAL DIAGNOSIS

LOOK FOR **additional traumatic** conditions for DRG 956, Limb reattachment, hip & femur proc for multiple significant trauma. If procedure performed for a diagnosis that is due to trauma, review for evidence of other significant trauma in **two or more** different body sites, e.g., traumatic brain injury, multiple rib fractures, etc.

Acute blood loss anemia due to the fracture and/or surgery is common. Review labs for drop in Hgb/Hct below normal or preop baseline. See *Acute Blood Loss Anemia*.

PROCEDURE

LOOK FOR diagnostic bone biopsy (ex. 0QB20ZX) performed during the hip procedure for DRGs 477-479, Biopsies of musculoskeletal system & connective tissue. Check operative note carefully and check for pathology report.

DRG 535	**Fractures of Hip & Pelvis w MCC**
DRG 536	**Fractures of Hip & Pelvis w/o MCC**

PRINCIPAL DIAGNOSIS

LOOK FOR osteoporosis as cause of fracture for DRGs 542-544, Path fxs & musc-skelet & conn tissue malignancy, when no surgical procedure performed. A diagnosis of osteoporosis = pathologic fracture (ex. M80.051A) if only minor trauma. See *Pathologic Fractures.*

PROCEDURE

LOOK FOR an operative procedure performed, such as ORIF for DRGs 480-482, Hip & femur proc, or hip replacement for DRGs 521-522, Hip replacement with principal diagnosis of hip fracture.

| DRG 551 | **Medical Back Problem w MCC** |
| DRG 552 | **Medical Back Problem w/o MCC** |

PRINCIPAL DIAGNOSIS

Elderly patients are frequently admitted for vertebral compression fractures. LOOK FOR a diagnosis of osteoporosis = pathologic fracture if only minor trauma for DRGs 542-544, Path fxs & musculoskeletal & connective tissue malig. See *Pathologic Fractures*.

Unspecified back pain alone is usually not sufficient to meet inpatient criteria, but may be treated in observation status to control pain. Inpatient admission is generally considered medically necessary for pathologic fracture.

LOOK FOR other possible causes of back pain, i.e., bowel obstruction, pancreatitis, shingles (H. zoster), gallbladder, kidney problems.

| DRG 557 | **Tendonitis, Myositis & Bursitis w MCC** |
| DRG 558 | **Tendonitis, Myositis & Bursitis w/o MCC** |

PRINCIPAL DIAGNOSIS

These DRGs include rhabdomyolysis (M62.82) assigned as principal diagnosis. For patients admitted with AKI/ATN due to rhabdomyolysis, the AKI/ATN would most likely be the principal diagnosis particularly if it was the focus of treatment for DRG 683, Renal failure w CC. See *Rhabdomyolysis*.

DRG 570-572 **Skin Debridement**

PRINCIPAL DIAGNOSIS

LOOK FOR evidence of "**necrotic**" tissue which is coded to gangrene (I96) if not elsewhere classified, with diabetes is coded E11.52 as principal diagnosis for DRG 264, Other circulatory system O.R. procedures.

LOOK FOR **diabetic** neuropathy (E11.40) or diabetic circulatory system (peripheral vascular) disease (E11.59) as cause of ulcer or cellulitis, which would assigned as the principal diagnosis for DRG 40-42, Peripheral/cranial nerve & other nervous system procedure, or DRG 264, Other circulatory system O.R. procedures.

LOOK FOR evidence of **cellulitis** (ex. L03.119) associated with skin ulcer. Cellulitis is unlikely to be principal diagnosis if excisional debridement performed for ulcer.

PROCEDURE
Verify that the procedure is "excisional". See *Excisional Debridement*.

DRG 579-581 Other Skin, Subcut Tissue & Breast Proc

PRINCIPAL DIAGNOSIS
LOOK FOR a diabetic complication as principal diagnosis when **toe amputation** performed, e.g., skin ulcer with DM (E11.622), osteomyelitis with DM (E11.69), for DRGs 616-618, Amputation of lower limb for endocrine, nutritional & metabolic disease.

DRG 592-594 Skin Ulcers

PRINCIPAL DIAGNOSIS
LOOK FOR clinical criteria for **sepsis** for DRGs 871-872, Septicemia or severe sepsis, in all patients with infection. See *Sepsis 2 or Sepsis 3*.

LOOK FOR evidence of **cellulitis** associated with skin ulcer for DRGs 602-603, Cellulitis. Sequencing depends upon focus of admission or may be co-equal. Cellulitis can usually be treated initially on an outpatient basis unless sepsis or other complication is present or failed outpatient treatment necessitates inpatient admission.

If patient admitted with both cellulitis and skin ulcer that are co-equal and there is no MCC, sequence skin ulcer as principal diagnosis; cellulitis would be CC. Cellulitis is unlikely to be principal diagnosis if excisional debridement performed. See *Skin/Pressure Ulcers.*

LOOK FOR evidence of cellulitis associated with skin ulcer.

LOOK FOR evidence of "**necrotic**" tissue. Necrotic/necrosis is coded as gangrene (I96) if not elsewhere classified; if with diabetes, code E11.52.

PROCEDURE

LOOK FOR for evidence of **"excisional" debridement** (excision, subcutaneous tissue and fascia) for DRGs 570-572, Skin debridement. Surgical removal or "cutting away" of devitalized subcutaneous tissue; use of term "excisional" is essential. See *Excisional Debridement.*

DRG 602	**Celluitis w MCC**
DRG 603	**Cellulitis w/o MCC**

PRINCIPAL DIAGNOSIS

Cellulitis can usually be treated initially on an outpatient basis unless sepsis or other complication is present, or failed outpatient treatment necessitates inpatient admission.

LOOK FOR clinical criteria for sepsis for DRGs 871-872, Sepsis. See *Sepsis 2 or Sepsis 3*.

If patient admitted with both cellulitis and skin ulcer that are co-equal and there is no MCC, sequence skin ulcer as principal diagnosis for DRGs 592-594, Skin ulcers. Cellulitis would be CC for principal diagnosis of skin ulcer. Cellulitis unlikely to be principal diagnosis if excisional debridement performed.

PROCEDURE

<u>LOOK FOR</u> evidence of **"excisional debridement"** or documentation of an **"excisional biopsy"** if abscess or skin ulcer present for DRGs 570-572, Skin debridement. Excisional debridement is the surgical removal or "cutting away" of devitalized tissue; use of term "excisional" is essential. An "excisional biopsy" of an abscess should be coded with a 7th digit of Z "no qualifier" when the abscess is completely excised, and should not be coded with 7th digit X for "diagnostic." For example, "excisional biopsy" of left thigh abscess which was completely excised is coded as 0JBM0ZZ. See *Excisional Debridement*.

An "incision and drainage" performed to surgically treat an abscess should be coded with 7th digit Z, rather than X "diagnostic" which is exclusively used for diagnostic procedures. For example, drainage of cutaneous abscess of the face to treat a facial abscess would be assigned code 0J910ZZ, for DRGs 137-138, Mouth Procedures.

| DRG 604 | **Trauma to the skin, subcut tissue & breast w MCC** |
| DRG 605 | **Trauma to the skin, subcut tissue & breast w/o MCC** |

PRINCIPAL DIAGNOSIS

<u>LOOK FOR</u> a more serious traumatic injury. For example, gun shot wound to the head coded as "puncture wound" or "open wound" of the head (S018- or S019-) are assigned to these DRGs which do not adequately describe this life-threatening injury.

GSW to head would usually be assigned to S062X- for traumatic diffuse intracranial or hemorrhagic brain injuries for DRGs 82-84, Traumatic stupor & coma, coma > 1 hr. When non-survivable injury and death, code S062X7A (diffuse traumatic brain injury w death). Code also any associated skull fracture, brain herniation, and/or brain death.

DRG 637-639 **Diabetes**

PRINCIPAL DIAGNOSIS

<u>LOOK FOR</u> associated diabetic **complications** such as:

- Gastroparesis (E11.43) or peripheral neuropathy (E11.40) for DRGs 73-74, Cranial or peripheral nerve disorders
- Circulatory/peripheral vascular disease (E11.59) for DRGs 299-301, Peripheral vascular disorders.

<u>LOOK FOR</u> alternative or co-equal diagnosis as principal reason for admission: dehydration, electrolyte imbalance, hyponatremia, hypokalemia, etc. for DRGs 640-641, Nutrition, metab, fluids/electrolyte dis. Determine the "focus" of the admission.

<u>LOOK FOR</u> hyperglycemia that is due to failure of insulin pump, in which case code T85.694A would be assigned as principal diagnosis for DRGs 919-921, Complications of treatment.

Chronic kidney disease (CKD) Stage 4 or 5 (N18.4, N18.5) is always a pertinent chronic condition and common in diabetes.

DRG 640   **Nutrition, Metab, Fluid/Elect Disorders w MCC**
DRG 641   **Nutrition, Metab, Fluid/Elect Disorders w/o MCC**

PRINCIPAL DIAGNOSIS

<u>LOOK FOR</u> criteria for **AKI** for DRG 682-684, Renal failure. Dehydration, commonly associated with electrolyte imbalance, is the most common cause of AKI. AKI is usually coded first in the presence of dehydration, since dehydration can often be treated in observation. However, sequencing of dehydration and AKI is based on the reason for the admission (CC 2019 Q1 p. 12). See *Acute Kidney Injury.*

<u>LOOK FOR</u> **SIADH** (E22.2) in patients with hyponatremia for DRGs 643-645, Endocrine disorders. See *Electrolyte Disorders*.

LOOK FOR **malignancy**. Patients admitted with an electrolyte imbalance due to a malignancy, code the electrolyte imbalance as principal diagnosis if admitted and treated for this only. If admission also includes any evaluation, treatment, or staging of a malignancy, the malignancy can be sequenced as the principal diagnosis.

LOOK FOR **fluid overload** due to heart failure for DRGs 291-293, Heart failure. Patients may be admitted for "fluid overload" when in reality they are also in CHF and treated for it. If CHF is documented it may be sequenced as principal diagnosis in this situation. See **Heart Failure**.

DRG 682-684 **Renal Failure**

PRINCIPAL DIAGNOSIS
Verify reason for admission and/or underlying etiology of AKI (if not due to dehydration), such as sepsis, acute MI, pneumonia as alternate principal diagnosis. When AKI is a manifestation of organ failure in septic patients, sepsis is sequenced first.

PROCEDURE
Review for procedure, i.e., dialysis AV shunt (ex. 031C0ZF), peritoneal fistula, or revision or removal of renal dialysis shunt (ex. 03PY07Z) for DRGs 673-675, Other kidney & urinary tract procedures.

DRG 689   **Kidney & Urinary Tract Infections w MCC**
DRG 690   **Kidney & Urinary Tract Infections w/o MCC**

PRINCIPAL DIAGNOSIS
Uncomplicated UTIs can usually be treated as an outpatient or in observation, in the absence of complications like sepsis, altered mental status (encephalopathy), acute kidney injury (AKI), multi-drug resistant organism, other.

LOOK FOR clinical criteria for **sepsis** for DRG 871-872, Sepsis. Many patients with UTI are actually admitted because they are septic. See *Sepsis-2* or *Sepsis-3* for clinical indicators.

LOOK FOR **encephalopathy** for DRGs 70-72, Nonspecific cerebrovascular disorders. Many patients with UTI, especially the elderly, will be admitted with altered mental status/encephalopathy which requires inpatient care. In this situation, encephalopathy should be diagnosed and sequenced as principal diagnosis when it is the cause of altered mental status. See *Encephalopathy*.

LOOK FOR **AKI** for DRGs 682-684, Renal failure. Patients with UTI are also frequently admitted because they are severely dehydrated and actually have AKI. Check for clinical criteria of AKI and sequence based on the circumstances/focus of admission. See *Acute Kidney Injury*.

LOOK FOR **infection due to Foley** (T83.511A) or other catheter for DRGs 698-700, Other kidney & urinary tract diagnoses. Must be specifically documented by the physician that the infection is "due to" the catheter or device. If not documented, a query to clarify is recommended. To be principal diagnosis the catheter must have been in place at or before the time of admission; make sure that a catheter was not inserted for the first time in the ED or on the unit.

| DRG 695 | **Kidney & Urin Tract Signs & Symptoms w MCC** |
| DRG 696 | **Kidney & Urin Tract Signs & Symptoms w/o MCC** |

PRINCIPAL DIAGNOSIS

Admission for symptoms such as urinary retention, hematuria, etc. is rarely needed unless a more complicated diagnosis is present or a procedure is performed.

LOOK FOR a more specific diagnosis rather than signs and symptoms such as UTI (DRGs 689-690), urinary stones (DRGs 693-694), urethral stricture (DRG 697). Signs and symptoms should not be used as a principal diagnosis if a possible/probable or confirmed cause is present.

| DRG 713 | **Transurethral Prostatectomy w MCC** |
| DRG 714 | **Transurethral Prostatectomy w/o MCC** |

PRINCIPAL DIAGNOSIS

TURP for BPH is usually performed on an outpatient basis.

<u>LOOK FOR</u> a **complication** or other condition as the reason for admission (principal diagnosis) following ambulatory surgery for DRGs 987-989, Non-extensive O.R. procedure unrelated to principal diagnosis. In these cases, the condition or complication such as postoperative bleeding, cardiac arrhythmia, ileus, atelectasis, etc. would be assigned as principal diagnosis and the surgical diagnosis as a secondary diagnosis. The surgical procedure is also coded.

If a patient is admitted with an **acute UTI** treated with antibiotics or for another acute urinary condition who subsequently has a TURP for the BPH, the principal diagnosis is assigned as UTI (or the other acute urinary condition), and the DRG becomes DRGs 665-667, "Prostatectomy [open]", not transurethral.

| DRG 749 | **Other Female Reprod System OR Proc w MCC** |
| DRG 750 | **Other Female Reprod System OR Proc w/o MCC** |

PRINCIPAL DIAGNOSIS

Determine whether postprocedural pelvic peritoneal adhesions (N99.4) vs. female pelvic adhesions (N73.6) is the principal diagnosis and reason for adhesiolysis (ex. 0DNW4ZZ) for DRGs 335-337, Peritoneal adhesiolysis.

| DRG 811 | **Anemia w MCC** |
| DRG 812 | **Anemia w/o MCC** |

PRINCIPAL DIAGNOSIS

LOOK FOR GI bleeding as cause of anemia for DRGs 377-379, G.I. hemorrhage. When patients are admitted for acute GI bleeding, the GI bleeding, or its cause, is nearly always sequenced as the principal diagnosis and acute blood loss anemia as a secondary diagnosis (CC). See *Acute Blood Loss Anemia*.

Per Coding Clinic, the combination codes for conditions such as ulcer, diverticulosis, diverticulitis, angiodysplasia, gastritis, esophagitis **"with" bleeding** or hemorrhage found during the diagnostic workup (colonoscopy, EGD) are assigned unless the provider documents a different cause of the bleeding or states that the conditions are unrelated.

Sometimes patients are admitted for chronic blood loss anemia due to chronic GI bleeding (known or unknown cause) and transfused. If there is no evaluation, treatment, or management directed at the chronic GI bleeding, the anemia is typically sequenced as principal diagnosis. The chronic GI bleeding (and its cause, if known) would then be a secondary diagnosis.

LOOK FOR **malignancy** associated with the anemia. When the admission is for management of an anemia associated with the malignancy, the malignancy is sequenced as the principal diagnosis. This rule does not apply to pancytopenia. See *Neoplasms*.

LOOK FOR **thrombocytopenia** for DRG 813, Coagulation disorders, or pancytopenia for DRGs 808–810, Major hematol/immun dx except sickle cell & coagul. Anemia in some patients is a part of their pancytopenia defined as neutropenia, thrombocytopenia, and anemia. When a diagnosis of pancytopenia is documented, it would become the principal diagnosis and anemia, thrombocytopenia, and neutropenia would not be separately coded. See *Pancytopenia*.

DRG 846-848 Chemotx w/o Acute Leukemia as SDX
DRG 849 Radiotherapy

PRINCIPAL DIAGNOSIS

If the patient is admitted solely for the purpose of receiving external beam radiotherapy, chemotherapy or immunotherapy, code Z51.0, Z51.11, or Z51.12 is sequenced as principal diagnosis. If one of these was not the sole reason for the admission but was also for workup, staging or other treatment of cancer, the malignancy could be sequenced as principal diagnosis.

If a patient admission is for the insertion or implantation of radioactive elements (e.g., brachytherapy), the appropriate code for the malignancy is sequenced as the principal or first-listed diagnosis. Code Z51.0 should not be assigned.

CC

LOOK FOR common comorbidities associated with malignancy which include metastases, pancytopenia, malnutrition, BMI < 20, major depression, AKI, pathologic fracture.

DRG 864 Fever and Inflammatory Conditions

PRINCIPAL DIAGNOSIS

DRG 864 includes fever (R50.9), drug-induced fever (R50.2), postprocedural fever (R50.82) which are all symptom codes and not assigned if explained by an underlying cause, especially infection. Also included in this DRG are the SIRS codes R65.10 and R65.11 which cannot be coded as a principal diagnosis.

LOOK FOR **sepsis** criteria in addition to fever for DRGs 871-872, Sepsis.

LOOK FOR **postop infection** (ex. T81.40XA) for DRGs 856-858, Postop & post-traumatic infections, i.e., admitted for possible infection causing fever following a surgical procedure, such as prostate biopsy.

LOOK FOR **viral illness** as etiology of fever for DRGs 865-866, Viral illness. Unspecified viral syndrome, code B34.9, would be used only when the type of virus has not been identified by laboratory tests and only when the symptom complex has not been identified, such as that of influenza (J11.1), viral hepatitis (B19.9), etc. Viral syndrome with associated diarrhea is assigned A08.4, viral enteritis.

LOOK FOR any indicators of a cause or possible/suspected cause of fever as a query opportunity. If no specific infection is identified and physician documentation indicates that an infection was suspected and treated (IV antibiotics), code to "**probable infection**" B99.9. A diagnosis of unspecified "bacterial infection" is coded A49.9. Both of these are assigned to DRGs 867-869, Other infectious and parasitic diseases dxs.

| DRG 871 | **Sepsis w/o Vent 96+ Hours w MCC** |
| DRG 872 | **Sepsis w/o Vent 96+ Hours w/o MCC** |

PRINCIPAL DIAGNOSIS

LOOK FOR **meningitis** as interrelated principal diagnosis for DRG 94, Bacterial & TB infections of nervous system. Most cases of meningitis are caused by bacteria or viruses that enter the bloodstream via the upper respiratory tract and then infect the meninges of the brain.

Meningitis is not typically a localized infection that progresses to sepsis. Bacteremia or septicemia, when it occurs, usually precedes the meningitis. Because there is no underlying/localized infection, the two may be considered interrelated and either sequenced as principal diagnosis, although meningitis is likely to be the focus of the admission.

LOOK FOR **sepsis** documented as **due to** (presence of) a cardiac or vascular device, implant, or graft for DRG 314, Other circulatory system diagnoses. A complication code would be coded as principal diagnosis.

LOOK FOR **sepsis due to Foley** (T83.511A) or other urinary catheter for DRG 698, Other kidney & urinary tract diagnoses w MCC, or other catheter such as PICC (T80.211A) or central line for DRG 314, Other circulatory system diagnoses w MCC. Provider documentation must indicate that the the infection is "due to" the catheter or device. If not documented, a query to clarify is recommended. To be principal diagnosis the catheter must have been in place at or before the time of admission; make sure that a catheter was not inserted for the first time in the ED or on the unit.

PROCEDURE

LOOK FOR evidence of an **operative procedure** performed in a patient with sepsis for DRG 853-855, Infectious & parasitic diseases w OR procedure, such as excisional debridement, transbronchial biopsy, or other significant procedure.

LOOK FOR **ventilator** 96+ hours. If patient on ventilator, follow and calculate duration carefully if longer than 96 hours for DRG 870, Sepsis w MV 96+ hours. See *Mechanical Ventilation* for calculation rules.

DRG 880   **Acute Adjust Reaction & Psychosocial Dysfunction**

PRINCIPAL DIAGNOSIS
Determine if acute anxiety, hostility, delirium, or hallucinations were possibly due to organic disturbances such as dementia (F03.90) or organic brain syndrome (F09) for DRG 884, Organic disturbances & mental retardation, or Alzheimer's disease (G30.9) for DRGs 56-57, Degenerative nervous system disorders. RX: Aricept, Exelon, Razadyne, Namenda, or anti-psychotics like Zyprexa, Geodon.

DRG 881   **Depressive Neuroses**
DRG 882   **Neuroses except Depressive**

PRINCIPAL DIAGNOSIS
LOOK FOR schizophrenia, bipolar disorder, or specified major depressive disorder as reason for admission for DRG 885, Psychoses.

DRG 896   **Alcohol/Drug Abuse or Dep w/o Rehab Tx w MCC**
DRG 897   **Alcohol/Drug Abuse or Dep w/o Rehab Tx w/o MCC**

PROCEDURE

<u>LOOK FOR</u> alcohol or drug rehabilitation (ex. HZ30ZZZ) provided for DRG 895, Alcohol/drug abuse or dependence with rehab therapy.

DRG 917   **Poisoning & Toxic Effect of Drugs w MCC**
DRG 918   **Poisoning & Toxic Effect of Drugs w/o MCC**

PRINCIPAL DIAGNOSIS

Confirm principal diagnosis is poisoning rather than an adverse effect. If adverse effect, assign the manifestation as the principal diagnosis, such as hypotension, arrhythmia, bleeding, AKI, rash, encephalopathy, etc. See *Adverse Reactions to Drugs & Toxins.*

DRG 919-921 **Complications of Treatment**

PRINCIPAL DIAGNOSIS

Confirm that the provider documentation indicates a cause-and-effect relationship between the condition and the care or procedure; however, there are many instances within the ICD-10 classification where the provider does not have to establish a causal relationship, e.g., surgical wound infection, postprocedural bleeding. See *Complications of Care.*

If the patient was admitted immediately following an outpatient procedure, assign the complication (or other reason for admission) as principal diagnosis. The condition for which the procedure was performed is assigned as a secondary diagnosis, and the surgical procedure is also coded.

DRG 947   **Signs & Symptoms w MCC**
DRG 948   **Signs & Symptoms w/o MCC**

PRINCIPAL DIAGNOSIS
These DRGs include malaise, pain, fatigue, mental status changes, and other conditions as principal diagnosis which are all symptom codes.

<u>LOOK FOR</u> cause or possible cause of symptoms, or other reasons for admission. Code first the cause. Do not code symptoms when more specific underlying (or probable) conditions are present. For example, ascites (R18.8) is a symptom code and is commonly caused by cirrhosis, malignancy, heart failure. See *Signs, Symptoms and Unspecified Codes.*

Patient should have "unstable" vital signs, abnormal lab or other significant clinical problems to meet criteria for inpatient admission; however, social admits may only have symptoms that can be appropriately assigned as principal diagnosis.

DRG 977   **HIV with or w/o Other Related Conditions**

<u>LOOK FOR</u> a "major related condition," which can be assigned as either principal or secondary diagnosis with code B20, for DRGs 974-976, HIV w major related condition. These include conditions such as candidiasis, thrush, psychosis, encephalopathy, herpes zoster/simplex, pneumonia, lymphoma, sepsis, etc. See *HIV/AIDS.*

DRG 981-983 **Extensive OR Proc Unrelated to PDX**
DRG 987-989 **Non-Extensive OR Proc Unrelated to PDX**

PRINCIPAL DIAGNOSIS

<u>LOOK FOR</u> a diagnosis "related" to the major surgical procedure as principal diagnosis to assign to a specific surgical DRG.

When these DRGs are assigned, always review the record carefully to determine whether the medical condition (or symptoms of the condition) associated with the principal surgical procedure might have been present on admission and could possibly meet the definition of principal diagnosis.

See further guidance at ***Unrelated OR Procedure DRGs*** in the Guidelines section.

S = Surgical DRG   M = Medical DRG   * = Post acute care transfer DRG   **GMLOS** = Geometric mean length of stay

DRG	Type	MS-DRG Title	Weight	GMLOS
1	S	Heart transplant or implant of heart assist system w MCC	28.9132	30.1
2	S	Heart transplant or implant of heart assist system w/o MCC	14.9701	15.4
3	S*	ECMO or trach w MV > 96 hrs or PDX exc face, mouth & neck w major O.R.	19.1055	22.4
4	S*	Trach w MV > 96 hrs or PDX exc face, mouth & neck w/o major O.R.	11.9225	20.0
5	S	Liver transplant w MCC or intestinal transplant	10.2350	14.4
6	S	Liver transplant w/o MCC	4.6964	7.5
7	S	Lung transplant	11.5800	17.4
8	S	Simultaneous pancreas/kidney transplant	5.4333	9.0
10	S	Pancreas transplant	3.6200	8.0
11	S	Tracheostomy for face, mouth & neck dxs or laryngectomy w MCC	5.0214	10.9
12	S	Tracheostomy for face, mouth & neck dxs or laryngectomy w CC	3.8328	8.3
13	S	Tracheostomy for face, mouth & neck dxs or laryngectomy w/o CC/MCC	2.7238	6.0
14	M	Allogeneic bone marrow transplant	10.6770	24.1
16	M	Autologous bone marrow transplant w CC/MCC	6.7363	17.1
17	M	Autologous bone marrow transplant w/o CC/MCC	4.8557	8.9
18	M	Chimeric Antigen Receptor (CAR) T-Cell and Other Immunotherapies	37.4501	15.6
19	S	Simultaneous Pancreas and Kidney Transplant with Hemodialysis	6.6797	11.0
20	S	Intracranial vascular procedures w PDX hemorrhage w MCC	10.3370	12.7
21	S	Intracranial vascular procedures w PDX hemorrhage w CC	7.5435	10.0
22	S	Intracranial vascular procedures w PDX hemorrhage w/o CC/MCC	4.8428	4.0

23	S*	Craniotomy w major device implant or acute complex CNS PDX w MCC or chemotherapy implant or epilepsy w neurostimulator	5.6719	7.1
24	S*	Craniotomy w major device implant or acute complex CNS PDX w/o MCC	3.9390	4.1
25	S*	Craniotomy & endovascular intracranial procedures w MCC	4.4974	6.6
26	S*	Craniotomy & endovascular intracranial procedures w CC	3.0620	3.8
27	S*	Craniotomy & endovascular intracranial procedures w/o CC/MCC	2.5143	1.9
28	S*	Spinal procedures w MCC	5.8231	9.3
29	S*	Spinal procedures w CC or spinal neurostimulators	3.2968	4.5
30	S*	Spinal procedures w/o CC/MCC	2.3568	2.4
31	S*	Ventricular shunt procedures w MCC	4.3717	7.2
32	S*	Ventricular shunt procedures w CC	2.2165	3.0
33	S*	Ventricular shunt procedures w/o CC/MCC	1.7222	1.7
34	S	Carotid artery stent procedure w MCC	3.9781	4.7
35	S	Carotid artery stent procedure w CC	2.3397	2.1
36	S	Carotid artery stent procedure w/o CC/MCC	1.8523	1.2
37	S	Extracranial procedures w MCC	3.2776	5.0
38	S	Extracranial procedures w CC	1.6588	2.1
39	S	Extracranial procedures w/o CC/MCC	1.1391	1.2
40	S*	Periph/cranial nerve & other nerv syst proc w MCC	3.8648	6.9
41	S*	Periph/cranial nerve & other nerv syst proc w CC or periph neurostim	2.3497	3.9
42	S*	Periph/cranial nerve & other nerv syst proc w/o CC/MCC	1.9012	2.4
52	M	Spinal disorders & injuries w CC/MCC	1.8535	4.2

53	M	Spinal disorders & injuries w/o CC/MCC	1.1364	2.8
54	M*	Nervous system neoplasms w MCC	1.3683	3.8
55	M*	Nervous system neoplasms w/o MCC	1.0446	3.0
56	M*	Degenerative nervous system disorders w MCC	2.1953	5.5
57	M*	Degenerative nervous system disorders w/o MCC	1.2675	3.9
58	M	Multiple sclerosis & cerebellar ataxia w MCC	1.7378	4.9
59	M	Multiple sclerosis & cerebellar ataxia w CC	1.1273	3.6
60	M	Multiple sclerosis & cerebellar ataxia w/o CC/MCC	0.9177	3.0
61	M	Ischemic stroke, precerebral occl or trans ischemia w TPA w MCC	2.8912	4.7
62	M	Ischemic stroke, precerebral occl or trans ischemia w TPA w CC	1.9883	3.2
63	M	Ischemic stroke, precerebral occl or trans ischemia w TPA w/o CC/MCC	1.7097	2.3
64	M*	Intracranial hemorrhage or cerebral infarction w MCC	1.9189	4.4
65	M*	Intracranial hemorrhage or cerebral infarction w CC or TPA in 24 hrs	1.0200	2.9
66	M*	Intracranial hemorrhage or cerebral infarction w/o CC/MCC	0.7116	2.0
67	M	Nonspecific CVA & precerebral occlusion w/o infarct w MCC	1.4258	3.3
68	M	Nonspecific CVA & precerebral occlusion w/o infarct w/o MCC	0.8889	2.1
69	M	Transient ischemia w/o thrombolytic	0.7871	2.1
70	M*	Nonspecific cerebrovascular disorders w MCC	1.6796	4.5
71	M*	Nonspecific cerebrovascular disorders w CC	1.0118	3.3
72	M*	Nonspecific cerebrovascular disorders w/o CC/MCC	0.7717	2.3
73	M	Cranial & peripheral nerve disorders w MCC	1.4529	3.7
74	M	Cranial & peripheral nerve disorders w/o MCC	1.0190	2.9

MS-DRG TABLE

75	M	Viral meningitis *w CC/MCC*	1.6270	4.7
76	M	Viral meningitis *w/o CC/MCC*	0.9849	3.0
77	M	Hypertensive encephalopathy *w MCC*	1.5329	4.0
78	M	Hypertensive encephalopathy *w CC*	0.9499	2.8
79	M	Hypertensive encephalopathy *w/o CC/MCC*	0.7288	2.0
80	M	Nontraumatic stupor & coma *w MCC*	2.0954	5.1
81	M	Nontraumatic stupor & coma *w/o MCC*	0.7732	2.5
82	M	Traumatic stupor & coma, coma >1 hr *w MCC*	2.2639	4.2
83	M	Traumatic stupor & coma, coma >1 hr *w CC*	1.3440	3.3
84	M	Traumatic stupor & coma, coma >1 hr *w/o CC/MCC*	0.9056	2.1
85	M*	Traumatic stupor & coma, coma <1 hr *w MCC*	2.3117	4.6
86	M*	Traumatic stupor & coma, coma <1 hr *w CC*	1.2745	3.0
87	M*	Traumatic stupor & coma, coma <1 hr *w/o CC/MCC*	0.8636	2.0
88	M	Concussion *w MCC*	1.4552	3.6
89	M	Concussion *w CC*	1.0635	2.7
90	M	Concussion *w/o CC/MCC*	0.8546	1.9
91	M*	Other disorders of nervous system *w MCC*	1.6508	4.2
92	M*	Other disorders of nervous system *w CC*	0.9889	3.0
93	M*	Other disorders of nervous system *w/o CC/MCC*	0.7822	2.2
94	M	Bacterial & tuberculous infections of nervous system *w MCC*	3.6379	8.0
95	M	Bacterial & tuberculous infections of nervous system *w CC*	2.5073	5.8
96	M	Bacterial & tuberculous infections of nervous system *w/o CC/MCC*	2.3327	4.2

97	M	Non-bacterial infect of nervous sys exc viral meningitis w MCC	3.7604	8.7
98	M	Non-bacterial infect of nervous sys exc viral meningitis w CC	2.1125	5.6
99	M	Non-bacterial infect of nervous sys exc viral meningitis w/o CC/MCC	1.4019	3.9
100	M*	Seizures w MCC	1.8764	4.3
101	M*	Seizures w/o MCC	0.8884	2.6
102	M	Headaches w MCC	1.1531	3.0
103	M	Headaches w/o MCC	0.8295	2.3
113	S	Orbital procedures w CC/MCC	2.1944	4.5
114	S	Orbital procedures w/o CC/MCC	1.4476	2.3
115	S	Extraocular procedures except orbit	1.4566	3.5
116	S	Intraocular procedures w CC/MCC	1.8827	4.1
117	S	Intraocular procedures w/o CC/MCC	1.0412	2.1
121	M	Acute major eye infections w CC/MCC	1.1906	4.2
122	M	Acute major eye infections w/o CC/MCC	0.6455	3.0
123	M	Neurological eye disorders	0.7668	2.0
124	M	Other disorders of the eye w MCC	1.4020	3.7
125	M	Other disorders of the eye w/o MCC	0.8370	2.5
135	S	Sinus & mastoid procedures w CC/MCC	2.1435	4.0
136	S	Sinus & mastoid procedures w/o CC/MCC	1.2555	1.6
137	S	Mouth procedures w CC/MCC	1.5097	3.7
138	S	Mouth procedures w/o CC/MCC	0.8565	1.9
139	S	Salivary gland procedures	1.2341	2.3

140	S	Major Head and Neck Procedures with MCC	3.9779	7.0
141	S	Major Head and Neck Procedures with CC	2.2061	3.3
142	S	Major Head and Neck Procedures without CC/MCC	1.6051	2.1
143	S	Other Ear, Nose, Mouth and Throat O.R. Procedures with MCC	2.9798	5.8
144	S	Other Ear, Nose, Mouth and Throat O.R. Procedures with CC	1.7615	3.1
145	S	Other Ear, Nose, Mouth and Throat O.R. Procedure without CC/MCC	1.2246	1.9
146	M	Ear, nose, mouth & throat malignancy *w MCC*	2.0411	5.1
147	M	Ear, nose, mouth & throat malignancy *w CC*	1.3011	3.4
148	M	Ear, nose, mouth & throat malignancy *w/o CC/MCC*	0.7870	2.2
149	M	Dysequilibrium	0.7370	2.0
150	M	Epistaxis *w MCC*	1.3275	3.4
151	M	Epistaxis *w/o MCC*	0.7384	2.1
152	M	Otitis media & URI *w MCC*	1.0805	3.1
153	M	Otitis media & URI *w/o MCC*	0.7132	2.3
154	M	Other ear, nose, mouth & throat diagnoses *w MCC*	1.5468	3.9
155	M	Other ear, nose, mouth & throat diagnoses *w CC*	0.9095	2.9
156	M	Other ear, nose, mouth & throat diagnoses *w/o CC/MCC*	0.6584	2.1
157	M	Dental & oral diseases *w MCC*	1.5762	4.3
158	M	Dental & oral diseases *w CC*	0.9002	2.8
159	M	Dental & oral diseases *w/o CC/MCC*	0.6631	2.1
163	S*	Major chest procedures *w MCC*	5.0068	9.2
164	S*	Major chest procedures *w CC*	2.6556	4.4

165	S*	Major chest procedures *w/o CC/MCC*	1.9166	2.6
166	S*	Other resp system O.R. procedures *w MCC*	3.7235	7.9
167	S*	Other resp system O.R. procedures *w CC*	1.8187	3.7
168	S*	Other resp system O.R. procedures *w/o CC/MCC*	1.3544	2.0
175	M*	Pulmonary embolism *w MCC or acute cor pulmonale*	1.5460	4.1
176	M*	Pulmonary embolism *w/o MCC*	0.8878	2.6
177	M*	Respiratory infections & inflammations *w MCC*	1.8491	5.4
178	M*	Respiratory infections & inflammations *w CC*	1.2078	4.0
179	M*	Respiratory infections & inflammations *w/o CC/MCC*	0.8727	3.0
180	M	Respiratory neoplasms *w MCC*	1.7399	4.9
181	M	Respiratory neoplasms *w CC*	1.1201	3.3
182	M	Respiratory neoplasms *w/o CC/MCC*	0.7920	2.2
183	M	Major chest trauma *w MCC*	1.5589	4.3
184	M	Major chest trauma *w CC*	1.0409	3.1
185	M	Major chest trauma *w/o CC/MCC*	0.7749	2.4
186	M*	Pleural effusion *w MCC*	1.5438	4.3
187	M*	Pleural effusion *w CC*	1.0329	3.2
188	M*	Pleural effusion *w/o CC/MCC*	0.7295	2.4
189	M	Pulmonary edema & respiratory failure	1.2261	3.6
190	M*	Chronic obstructive pulmonary disease *w MCC*	1.1251	3.6
191	M*	Chronic obstructive pulmonary disease *w CC*	0.8843	2.9
192	M*	Chronic obstructive pulmonary disease *w/o CC/MCC*	0.6956	2.4

193	M*	Simple pneumonia & pleurisy w MCC	1.3120	4.1
194	M*	Simple pneumonia & pleurisy w CC	0.8639	3.1
195	M*	Simple pneumonia & pleurisy w/o CC/MCC	0.6658	2.5
196	M*	Interstitial lung disease w MCC	1.7386	4.8
197	M*	Interstitial lung disease w CC	1.0070	3.2
198	M*	Interstitial lung disease w/o CC/MCC	0.7434	2.4
199	M	Pneumothorax w MCC	1.7900	5.1
200	M	Pneumothorax w CC	1.0765	3.2
201	M	Pneumothorax w/o CC/MCC	0.7096	2.3
202	M	Bronchitis & asthma w CC/MCC	0.9670	3.0
203	M	Bronchitis & asthma w/o CC/MCC	0.7070	2.3
204	M	Respiratory signs & symptoms	0.7936	2.1
205	M*	Other respiratory system diagnoses w MCC	1.6848	4.1
206	M*	Other respiratory system diagnoses w/o MCC	0.8860	2.5
207	M*	Respiratory system diagnosis w ventilator support >96 hours	5.7361	11.9
208	M	Respiratory system diagnosis w ventilator support <=96 hours	2.5448	4.9
215	S	Other heart assist system implant	10.5584	5.1
216	S*	Cardiac valve & oth maj cardiothoracic proc w card cath w MCC	10.0393	11.6
217	S*	Cardiac valve & oth maj cardiothoracic proc w card cath w CC	6.4835	6.2
218	S*	Cardiac valve & oth maj cardiothoracic proc w card cath w/o CC/MCC	6.1093	3.1
219	S*	Cardiac valve & oth maj cardiothoracic proc w/o card cath w MCC	8.0576	8.9
220	S*	Cardiac valve & oth maj cardiothoracic proc w/o card cath w CC	5.4053	5.9

221	S*	Cardiac valve & oth maj cardiothoracic proc w/o card cath w/o CC/MCC	4.5799	3.8
222	S	Cardiac defib implant w cardiac cath w AMI/HF/shock w MCC	7.9510	8.8
223	S	Cardiac defib implant w cardiac cath w AMI/HF/shock w/o MCC	5.7986	4.7
224	S	Cardiac defib implant w cardiac cath w/o AMI/HF/shock w MCC	7.5191	7.6
225	S	Cardiac defib implant w cardiac cath w/o AMI/HF/shock w/o MCC	5.6178	4.2
226	S	Cardiac defibrillator implant w/o cardiac cath w MCC	6.5650	6.1
227	S	Cardiac defibrillator implant w/o cardiac cath w/o MCC	5.2121	3.0
228	S	Other cardiothoracic procedures w MCC	5.3303	7.0
229	S	Other cardiothoracic procedures w/o MCC	3.4412	3.0
231	S	Coronary bypass w PTCA w MCC	8.7159	10.8
232	S	Coronary bypass w PTCA w/o MCC	5.9538	7.7
233	S*	Coronary bypass w cardiac cath w MCC	7.9223	11.4
234	S*	Coronary bypass w cardiac cath w/o MCC	5.3360	8.1
235	S*	Coronary bypass w/o cardiac cath w MCC	6.1041	8.6
236	S*	Coronary bypass w/o cardiac cath w/o MCC	4.0970	6.0
239	S*	Amputation for circ sys disorders exc upper limb & toe w MCC	4.8160	10.4
240	S*	Amputation for circ sys disorders exc upper limb & toe w CC	2.7888	7.0
241	S*	Amputation for circ sys disorders exc upper limb & toe w/o CC/MCC	1.5924	4.4
242	S*	Permanent cardiac pacemaker implant w MCC	3.7276	5.2
243	S*	Permanent cardiac pacemaker implant w CC	2.5185	3.1
244	S*	Permanent cardiac pacemaker implant w/o CC/MCC	2.0633	2.2
245	S	AICD generator procedures	5.4178	4.7

246	S	Perc cardiovasc proc w drug-eluting stent w MCC or 4+ arteries or stents	3.1243	3.9
247	S	Perc cardiovasc proc w drug-eluting stent w/o MCC	1.9732	2.1
248	S	Perc cardiovasc proc w non-drug-eluting stent w MCC or 4+ arteries or stents	3.1622	4.5
249	S	Perc cardiovasc proc w non-drug-eluting stent w/o MCC	1.8737	2.2
250	S	Perc cardiovasc proc w/o coronary artery stent w MCC	2.5218	3.7
251	S	Perc cardiovasc proc w/o coronary artery stent w/o MCC	1.6584	2.1
252	S	Other vascular procedures w MCC	3.3257	5.2
253	S	Other vascular procedures w CC	2.6536	4.0
254	S	Other vascular procedures w/o CC/MCC	1.8159	2.1
255	S*	Upper limb & toe amputation for circ system disorders w MCC	2.5353	6.5
256	S*	Upper limb & toe amputation for circ system disorders w CC	1.6442	5.0
257	S*	Upper limb & toe amputation for circ system disorders w/o CC/MCC	1.1652	3.5
258	S	Cardiac pacemaker device replacement w MCC	3.1681	5.0
259	S	Cardiac pacemaker device replacement w/o MCC	2.0892	2.6
260	S	Cardiac pacemaker revision except device replacement w MCC	3.5673	6.4
261	S	Cardiac pacemaker revision except device replacement w CC	1.9939	3.2
262	S	Cardiac pacemaker revision except device replacement w/o CC/MCC	1.7062	2.2
263	S	Vein ligation & stripping	2.3132	4.4
264	S*	Other circulatory system O.R. procedures	3.2536	6.5
265	S	AICD lead procedures	3.3655	3.7
266	S*	Endovascular cardiac valve replacement & supplement procs w MCC	7.0479	3.2
267	S*	Endovascular cardiac valve replacement & supplement procs w/o MCC	5.5980	1.7

268	S	Aortic and heart assist procedures except pulsation balloon w MCC	6.9633	6.3
269	S	Aortic and heart assist procedures except pulsation balloon w/o MCC	4.3151	1.6
270	S	Other major cardiovascular procedures w MCC	5.1870	6.6
271	S	Other major cardiovascular procedures w CC	3.5654	4.3
272	S	Other major cardiovascular procedures w/o CC/MCC	2.6883	2.0
273	S*	Percutaneous intracardiac procedures w MCC	3.8267	4.3
274	S*	Percutaneous intracardiac procedures w/o MCC	3.2866	1.5
280	M*	Acute myocardial infarction, discharged alive w MCC	1.6069	4.1
281	M*	Acute myocardial infarction, discharged alive w CC	0.9306	2.5
282	M*	Acute myocardial infarction, discharged alive w/o CC/MCC	0.7261	1.8
283	M	Acute myocardial infarction, expired w MCC	1.8647	2.9
284	M	Acute myocardial infarction, expired w CC	0.7234	1.6
285	M	Acute myocardial infarction, expired w/o CC/MCC	0.4947	1.2
286	M	Circulatory disorders except AMI, w card cath w MCC	2.1363	5.2
287	M	Circulatory disorders except AMI, w card cath w/o MCC	1.1151	2.2
288	M*	Acute & subacute endocarditis w MCC	2.6854	7.1
289	M*	Acute & subacute endocarditis w CC	1.6436	5.3
290	M*	Acute & subacute endocarditis w/o CC/MCC	1.0269	3.6
291	M*	Heart failure & shock w MCC	1.2683	3.8
292	M*	Heart failure & shock w CC	0.8635	3.0
293	M*	Heart failure & shock w/o CC/MCC	0.5899	2.2
294	M	Deep vein thrombophlebitis w CC/MCC	1.2828	3.3

295	M	Deep vein thrombophlebitis w/o CC/MCC	0.9841	2.6
296	M	Cardiac arrest, unexplained w MCC	1.5952	2.0
297	M	Cardiac arrest, unexplained w CC	0.7070	1.3
298	M	Cardiac arrest, unexplained w/o CC/MCC	0.4888	1.1
299	M*	Peripheral vascular disorders w MCC	1.5326	3.9
300	M*	Peripheral vascular disorders w CC	1.0438	3.1
301	M*	Peripheral vascular disorders w/o CC/MCC	0.7431	2.2
302	M	Atherosclerosis w MCC	1.0948	2.7
303	M	Atherosclerosis w/o MCC	0.6776	1.9
304	M	Hypertension w MCC	1.0970	2.9
305	M	Hypertension w/o MCC	0.7399	2.2
306	M	Cardiac congenital & valvular disorders w MCC	1.5074	3.7
307	M	Cardiac congenital & valvular disorders w/o MCC	0.8704	2.4
308	M	Cardiac arrhythmia & conduction disorders w MCC	1.2009	3.5
309	M	Cardiac arrhythmia & conduction disorders w CC	0.7505	2.4
310	M	Cardiac arrhythmia & conduction disorders w/o CC/MCC	0.5592	1.9
311	M	Angina pectoris	0.6985	1.9
312	M	Syncope & collapse	0.8387	2.3
313	M	Chest pain	0.7214	1.7
314	M*	Other circulatory system diagnoses w MCC	2.0847	4.8
315	M*	Other circulatory system diagnoses w CC	0.9734	2.8
316	M*	Other circulatory system diagnoses w/o CC/MCC	0.7234	1.9

319	S	Other endovascular cardiac valve procedures w MCC	4.3179	7.7
320	S	Other endovascular cardiac valve procedures w/o MCC	2.4056	2.4
326	S*	Stomach, esophageal & duodenal proc w MCC	5.3163	9.5
327	S*	Stomach, esophageal & duodenal proc w CC	2.5647	4.6
328	S*	Stomach, esophageal & duodenal proc w/o CC/MCC	1.6669	2.3
329	S*	Major small & large bowel procedures w MCC	4.8862	10.3
330	S*	Major small & large bowel procedures w CC	2.5493	5.7
331	S*	Major small & large bowel procedures w/o CC/MCC	1.7105	3.3
332	S*	Rectal resection w MCC	4.1615	7.9
333	S*	Rectal resection w CC	2.1413	4.1
334	S*	Rectal resection w/o CC/MCC	1.6086	2.5
335	S*	Peritoneal adhesiolysis w MCC	3.9135	9.3
336	S*	Peritoneal adhesiolysis w CC	2.2913	5.9
337	S*	Peritoneal adhesiolysis w/o CC/MCC	1.6373	3.7
338	S	Appendectomy w complicated principal diag w MCC	2.7973	6.4
339	S	Appendectomy w complicated principal diag w CC	1.6974	4.0
340	S	Appendectomy w complicated principal diag w/o CC/MCC	1.2283	2.4
341	S	Appendectomy w/o complicated principal diag w MCC	2.3224	4.3
342	S	Appendectomy w/o complicated principal diag w CC	1.4329	2.7
343	S	Appendectomy w/o complicated principal diag w/o CC/MCC	1.1086	1.7
344	S	Minor small & large bowel procedures w MCC	2.8184	7.0
345	S	Minor small & large bowel procedures w CC	1.5788	4.3

346	S	Minor small & large bowel procedures w/o CC/MCC	1.2754	3.1
347	S	Anal & stomal procedures w MCC	2.4647	5.6
348	S	Anal & stomal procedures w CC	1.3481	3.3
349	S	Anal & stomal procedures w/o CC/MCC	0.9793	1.9
350	S	Inguinal & femoral hernia procedures w MCC	2.4548	5.2
351	S	Inguinal & femoral hernia procedures w CC	1.4927	3.2
352	S	Inguinal & femoral hernia procedures w/o CC/MCC	1.1044	2.0
353	S	Hernia procedures except inguinal & femoral w MCC	3.0249	5.9
354	S	Hernia procedures except inguinal & femoral w CC	1.7848	3.6
355	S	Hernia procedures except inguinal & femoral w/o CC/MCC	1.3602	2.4
356	S*	Other digestive system O.R. procedures w MCC	4.3078	7.7
357	S*	Other digestive system O.R. procedures w CC	2.2685	4.6
358	S*	Other digestive system O.R. procedures w/o CC/MCC	1.3491	2.8
368	M	Major esophageal disorders w MCC	1.9491	4.6
369	M	Major esophageal disorders w CC	1.0772	3.1
370	M	Major esophageal disorders w/o CC/MCC	0.7481	2.1
371	M*	Major GI disorders & peritoneal infections w MCC	1.7312	5.2
372	M*	Major GI disorders & peritoneal infections w CC	1.0293	3.8
373	M*	Major GI disorders & peritoneal infections w/o CC/MCC	0.7446	2.9
374	M*	Digestive malignancy w MCC	2.0737	5.5
375	M*	Digestive malignancy w CC	1.2076	3.6
376	M*	Digestive malignancy w/o CC/MCC	0.8989	2.5

377	M*	G.I. hemorrhage *w MCC*	1.8012	4.4
378	M*	G.I. hemorrhage *w CC*	0.9935	3.0
379	M*	G.I. hemorrhage *w/o CC/MCC*	0.6372	2.1
380	M*	Complicated peptic ulcer *w MCC*	1.8866	4.9
381	M*	Complicated peptic ulcer *w CC*	1.0593	3.2
382	M*	Complicated peptic ulcer *w/o CC/MCC*	0.7686	2.4
383	M	Uncomplicated peptic ulcer *w MCC*	1.3126	3.8
384	M	Uncomplicated peptic ulcer *w/o MCC*	0.8928	2.5
385	M	Inflammatory bowel disease *w MCC*	1.6223	5.0
386	M	Inflammatory bowel disease *w CC*	0.9951	3.5
387	M	Inflammatory bowel disease *w/o CC/MCC*	0.7147	2.6
388	M*	G.I. obstruction *w MCC*	1.5146	4.7
389	M*	G.I. obstruction *w CC*	0.8232	3.2
390	M*	G.I. obstruction *w/o CC/MCC*	0.5831	2.4
391	M	Esophagitis, gastroent & misc digest disorders *w MCC*	1.2492	3.7
392	M	Esophagitis, gastroent & misc digest disorders *w/o MCC*	0.7658	2.6
393	M	Other digestive system diagnoses *w MCC*	1.6612	4.3
394	M	Other digestive system diagnoses *w CC*	0.9409	3.0
395	M	Other digestive system diagnoses *w/o CC/MCC*	0.6515	2.2
405	S*	Pancreas, liver & shunt procedures *w MCC*	5.7376	9.5
406	S*	Pancreas, liver & shunt procedures *w CC*	2.8809	5.1
407	S*	Pancreas, liver & shunt procedures *w/o CC/MCC*	2.1180	3.7

408	S	Biliary tract proc except only cholecyst w or w/o C.D.E. w MCC	3.7529	8.5
409	S	Biliary tract proc except only cholecyst w or w/o C.D.E. w CC	2.1164	4.8
410	S	Biliary tract proc except only cholecyst w or w/o C.D.E. w/o CC/MCC	1.5683	3.5
411	S	Cholecystectomy w C.D.E. w MCC	3.7535	7.8
412	S	Cholecystectomy w C.D.E. w CC	2.2775	5.0
413	S	Cholecystectomy w C.D.E. w/o CC/MCC	1.7309	3.6
414	S*	Cholecystectomy except by laparoscope w/o C.D.E. w MCC	3.6283	8.0
415	S*	Cholecystectomy except by laparoscope w/o C.D.E. w CC	2.0317	4.9
416	S*	Cholecystectomy except by laparoscope w/o C.D.E. w/o CC/MCC	1.4223	3.0
417	S	Laparoscopic cholecystectomy w/o C.D.E. w MCC	2.4243	5.1
418	S	Laparoscopic cholecystectomy w/o C.D.E. w CC	1.6890	3.5
419	S	Laparoscopic cholecystectomy w/o C.D.E. w/o CC/MCC	1.3153	2.4
420	S	Hepatobiliary diagnostic procedures w MCC	3.5165	7.3
421	S	Hepatobiliary diagnostic procedures w CC	1.9075	3.8
422	S	Hepatobiliary diagnostic procedures w/o CC/MCC	1.4536	2.7
423	S	Other hepatobiliary or pancreas O.R. procedures w MCC	4.1859	8.4
424	S	Other hepatobiliary or pancreas O.R. procedures w CC	2.2841	4.7
425	S	Other hepatobiliary or pancreas O.R. procedures w/o CC/MCC	1.5427	2.2
432	M	Cirrhosis & alcoholic hepatitis w MCC	1.8808	4.7
433	M	Cirrhosis & alcoholic hepatitis w CC	1.0299	3.3
434	M	Cirrhosis & alcoholic hepatitis w/o CC/MCC	0.6207	2.2
435	M	Malignancy of hepatobiliary system or pancreas w MCC	1.7534	4.8

436	M	Malignancy of hepatobiliary system or pancreas *w CC*	1.1215	3.4
437	M	Malignancy of hepatobiliary system or pancreas *w/o CC/MCC*	0.8959	2.4
438	M	Disorders of pancreas except malignancy *w MCC*	1.5978	4.6
439	M	Disorders of pancreas except malignancy *w CC*	0.8452	3.1
440	M	Disorders of pancreas except malignancy *w/o CC/MCC*	0.6063	2.4
441	M*	Disorders of liver except malig, cirr, alc hepa *w MCC*	1.8795	4.7
442	M*	Disorders of liver except malig, cirr, alc hepa *w CC*	0.9300	3.2
443	M*	Disorders of liver except malig, cirr, alc hepa *w/o CC/MCC*	0.6632	2.4
444	M	Disorders of the biliary tract *w MCC*	1.6716	4.4
445	M	Disorders of the biliary tract *w CC*	1.0775	3.0
446	M	Disorders of the biliary tract *w/o CC/MCC*	0.8166	2.2
453	S	Combined anterior/posterior spinal fusion *w MCC*	9.1880	7.5
454	S	Combined anterior/posterior spinal fusion *w CC*	6.0931	3.8
455	S	Combined anterior/posterior spinal fusion *w/o CC/MCC*	4.7813	2.4
456	S	Spinal fus exc cerv *w spinal curv/malig/infec or ext fus w MCC*	8.6000	9.5
457	S	Spinal fus exc cerv *w spinal curv/malig/infec or ext fus w CC*	6.4959	5.2
458	S	Spinal fus exc cerv *w spinal curv/malig/infec or ext fus w/o CC/MCC*	5.0076	3.0
459	S*	Spinal fusion except cervical *w MCC*	6.7335	6.9
460	S*	Spinal fusion except cervical *w/o MCC*	3.9307	2.7
461	S	Bilateral or multiple major joint procs of lower extremity *w MCC*	6.0817	6.7
462	S	Bilateral or multiple major joint procs of lower extremity *w/o MCC*	3.1414	2.6
463	S*	Wnd debrid & skn grft exc hand for musculo-conn tiss dis *w MCC*	5.3703	9.9

464	S*	Wnd debrid & skn grft exc hand for musculo-conn tiss dis w CC	2.9759	5.5
465	S*	Wnd debrid & skn grft exc hand for musculo-conn tiss dis w/o CC/MCC	1.8441	2.6
466	S*	Revision of hip or knee replacement w MCC	5.3457	7.0
467	S*	Revision of hip or knee replacement w CC	3.5775	3.3
468	S*	Revision of hip or knee replacement w/o CC/MCC	2.8024	1.9
469	S*	Major hip/knee joint replacement or reattachment of lower extremity w MCC or total ankle replacement	3.0859	3.1
470	S*	Major hip/knee joint replacement or reattachment of lower extremity w/o MCC	1.9003	1.8
471	S	Cervical spinal fusion w MCC	5.0197	6.8
472	S	Cervical spinal fusion w CC	3.0537	2.5
473	S	Cervical spinal fusion w/o CC/MCC	2.5390	1.6
474	S*	Amputation for musculoskeletal sys & conn tissue dis w MCC	4.0761	9.4
475	S*	Amputation for musculoskeletal sys & conn tissue dis w CC	2.1963	5.8
476	S*	Amputation for musculoskeletal sys & conn tissue dis w/o CC/MCC	1.1603	2.9
477	S*	Biopsies of musculoskeletal system & connective tissue w MCC	3.3589	8.1
478	S*	Biopsies of musculoskeletal system & connective tissue w CC	2.3584	5.2
479	S*	Biopsies of musculoskeletal system & connective tissue w/o CC/MCC	1.8095	3.3
480	S*	Hip & femur procedures except major joint w MCC	3.0258	6.2
481	S*	Hip & femur procedures except major joint w CC	2.0961	4.3
482	S*	Hip & femur procedures except major joint w/o CC/MCC	1.6458	3.3
483	S	Major joint/limb reattachment proc of upper extremities	2.3857	1.4

485	S	Knee procedures w pdx of infection w MCC	3.4096	8.0
486	S	Knee procedures w pdx of infection w CC	2.1494	5.2
487	S	Knee procedures w pdx of infection w/o CC/MCC	1.6402	3.6
488	S*	Knee procedures w/o pdx of infection w CC/MCC	1.9757	3.1
489	S*	Knee procedures w/o pdx of infection w/o CC/MCC	1.2982	1.7
492	S*	Lower extrem & humer proc except hip, foot, femur w MCC	3.4700	6.2
493	S*	Lower extrem & humer proc except hip, foot, femur w CC	2.3258	4.0
494	S*	Lower extrem & humer proc except hip, foot, femur w/o CC/MCC	1.8517	2.7
495	S*	Local excision & removal int fix devices exc hip & femur w MCC	3.6419	7.3
496	S*	Local excision & removal int fix devices exc hip & femur w CC	1.9864	3.4
497	S*	Local excision & removal int fix devices exc hip & femur w/o CC/MCC	1.4515	1.8
498	S	Local excision & removal int fix devices of hip & femur w CC/MCC	2.5837	5.6
499	S	Local excision & removal int fix devices of hip & femur w/o CC/MCC	1.1990	2.0
500	S*	Soft tissue procedures w MCC	3.1895	7.4
501	S*	Soft tissue procedures w CC	1.7541	4.1
502	S*	Soft tissue procedures w/o CC/MCC	1.3328	2.4
503	S	Foot procedures w MCC	2.6406	6.8
504	S	Foot procedures w CC	1.7750	4.0
505	S	Foot procedures w/o CC/MCC	1.7750	4.0
506	S	Major thumb or joint procedures	1.4836	3.9
507	S	Major shoulder or elbow joint procedures w CC/MCC	2.0609	4.7
508	S	Major shoulder or elbow joint procedures w/o CC/MCC	1.4097	2.3

509	S	Arthroscopy	1.6865	4.1
510	S*	Shoulder, elbow or forearm proc, exc major joint proc w MCC	2.7437	4.9
511	S*	Shoulder, elbow or forearm proc, exc major joint proc w CC	1.9674	3.4
512	S*	Shoulder, elbow or forearm proc, exc major joint proc w/o CC/MCC	1.5545	2.1
513	S	Hand or wrist proc, except major thumb or joint proc w CC/MCC	1.5720	4.0
514	S	Hand or wrist proc, except major thumb or joint proc w/o CC/MCC	0.9991	2.4
515	S*	Other musculoskelet sys & conn tiss O.R. proc w MCC	3.1406	6.4
516	S*	Other musculoskelet sys & conn tiss O.R. proc w CC	1.9628	3.7
517	S*	Other musculoskelet sys & conn tiss O.R. proc w/o CC/MCC	1.3982	2.1
518	S*	Back & neck proc exc spinal fusion w MCC or disc device/neurostim	3.5869	4.2
519	S*	Back & neck proc exc spinal fusion w CC	1.9600	3.2
520	S*	Back & neck proc exc spinal fusion w/o CC/MCC	1.4183	2.0
521	S*	Hip Replacement with Principal Diagnosis of Hip Fracture with MCC	3.0662	6.2
522	S*	Hip Replacement with Principal Diagnosis of Hip Fracture without MCC	2.1894	4.1
533	M*	Fractures of femur w MCC	1.4162	4.0
534	M*	Fractures of femur w/o MCC	0.7902	2.8
535	M*	Fractures of hip & pelvis w MCC	1.2328	3.8
536	M*	Fractures of hip & pelvis w/o MCC	0.7717	2.9
537	M	Sprains, strains, & dislocations of hip, pelvis & thigh w CC/MCC	0.9354	3.1
538	M	Sprains, strains, & dislocations of hip, pelvis & thigh w/o CC/MCC	0.7232	2.6
539	M*	Osteomyelitis w MCC	1.9477	5.9
540	M*	Osteomyelitis w CC	1.3016	4.3

541	M*	Osteomyelitis w/o CC/MCC	0.8432	3.1
542	M*	Pathological fractures & musculoskelet & conn tiss malig w MCC	1.8092	5.0
543	M*	Pathological fractures & musculoskelet & conn tiss malig w CC	1.0452	3.5
544	M*	Pathological fractures & musculoskelet & conn tiss malig w/o CC/MCC	0.7777	2.8
545	M*	Connective tissue disorders w MCC	2.5031	5.5
546	M*	Connective tissue disorders w CC	1.2080	3.5
547	M*	Connective tissue disorders w/o CC/MCC	0.8336	2.5
548	M	Septic arthritis w MCC	2.0508	5.7
549	M	Septic arthritis w CC	1.2499	4.0
550	M	Septic arthritis w/o CC/MCC	0.8789	3.0
551	M*	Medical back problems w MCC	1.6274	4.3
552	M*	Medical back problems w/o MCC	0.9434	2.9
553	M	Bone diseases & arthropathies w MCC	1.2715	3.9
554	M	Bone diseases & arthropathies w/o MCC	0.7925	2.8
555	M	Signs & symptoms of musculoskeletal system & conn tissue w MCC	1.3685	3.8
556	M	Signs & symptoms of musculoskeletal system & conn tissue w/o MCC	0.8087	2.6
557	M*	Tendonitis, myositis & bursitis w MCC	1.3991	4.6
558	M*	Tendonitis, myositis & bursitis w/o MCC	0.8614	3.1
559	M*	Aftercare, musculoskeletal system & connective tissue w MCC	1.8653	4.9
560	M*	Aftercare, musculoskeletal system & connective tissue w CC	1.0760	3.7
561	M*	Aftercare, musculoskeletal system & connective tissue w/o CC/MCC	0.7924	2.7
562	M*	Fx, sprn, strn & disloc except femur, hip, pelvis & thigh w MCC	1.4118	4.0

MS-DRG TABLE

563	M*	Fx, sprn, strn & disl except femur, hip, pelvis & thigh w/o MCC	0.8722	3.0
564	M	Other musculoskeletal sys & connective tissue diagnoses w MCC	1.5236	4.6
565	M	Other musculoskeletal sys & connective tissue diagnoses w CC	1.0093	3.4
566	M	Other musculoskeletal sys & connective tissue diagnoses w/o CC/MCC	0.7519	2.5
570	S*	Skin debridement w MCC	2.8417	7.3
571	S*	Skin debridement w CC	1.6354	4.8
572	S*	Skin debridement w/o CC/MCC	1.1044	3.0
573	S*	Skin graft for skin ulcer or cellulitis w MCC	5.5391	10.8
574	S*	Skin graft for skin ulcer or cellulitis w CC	3.2465	7.6
575	S*	Skin graft for skin ulcer or cellulitis w/o CC/MCC	1.7632	4.5
576	S	Skin graft except for skin ulcer or cellulitis w MCC	5.0637	9.3
577	S	Skin graft except for skin ulcer or cellulitis w CC	2.5496	4.6
578	S	Skin graft except for skin ulcer or cellulitis w/o CC/MCC	1.5952	2.8
579	S*	Other skin, subcut tiss & breast proc w MCC	3.1449	7.3
580	S*	Other skin, subcut tiss & breast proc w CC	1.7288	4.1
581	S*	Other skin, subcut tiss & breast proc w/o CC/MCC	1.3768	2.2
582	S	Mastectomy for malignancy w CC/MCC	1.6431	2.3
583	S	Mastectomy for malignancy w/o CC/MCC	1.5415	1.7
584	S	Breast biopsy, local excision & other breast procedures w CC/MCC	1.8367	3.5
585	S	Breast biopsy, local excision & other breast procedures w/o CC/MCC	1.7396	2.2
592	M*	Skin ulcers w MCC	1.6943	5.4
593	M*	Skin ulcers w CC	1.1406	4.1

594	M*	Skin ulcers w/o CC/MCC	0.8160	3.2
595	M	Major skin disorders w MCC	2.0165	5.5
596	M	Major skin disorders w/o MCC	0.9947	3.3
597	M	Malignant breast disorders w MCC	1.6440	4.6
598	M	Malignant breast disorders w CC	1.1129	3.3
599	M	Malignant breast disorders w/o CC/MCC	0.6714	2.5
600	M	Non-malignant breast disorders w CC/MCC	0.9969	3.5
601	M	Non-malignant breast disorders w/o CC/MCC	0.6868	2.8
602	M*	Cellulitis w MCC	1.4500	4.6
603	M*	Cellulitis w/o MCC	0.8536	3.2
604	M	Trauma to the skin, subcut tiss & breast w MCC	1.4779	3.8
605	M	Trauma to the skin, subcut tiss & breast w/o MCC	0.9039	2.7
606	M	Minor skin disorders w MCC	1.5121	4.3
607	M	Minor skin disorders w/o MCC	0.8282	2.9
614	S	Adrenal & pituitary procedures w CC/MCC	2.3897	3.2
615	S	Adrenal & pituitary procedures w/o CC/MCC	1.5750	1.8
616	S*	Amputat of lower limb for endocrine, nutrit, & metabol dis w MCC	3.9662	10.0
617	S*	Amputat of lower limb for endocrine, nutrit, & metabol dis w CC	2.0298	5.8
618	S*	Amputat of lower limb for endocrine, nutrit, & metabol dis w/o CC/MCC	1.3032	4.2
619	S	O.R. procedures for obesity w MCC	3.0617	2.8
620	S	O.R. procedures for obesity w CC	1.7627	1.8
621	S	O.R. procedures for obesity w/o CC/MCC	1.5971	1.4

622	S*	Skin grafts & wound debrid for endoc, nutrit & metab dis w MCC	3.6149	8.3
623	S*	Skin grafts & wound debrid for endoc, nutrit & metab dis w CC	1.8715	5.3
624	S*	Skin grafts & wound debrid for endoc, nutrit & metab dis w/o CC/MCC	1.0989	3.2
625	S	Thyroid, parathyroid & thyroglossal procedures w MCC	2.8402	4.8
626	S	Thyroid, parathyroid & thyroglossal procedures w CC	1.6529	2.3
627	S	Thyroid, parathyroid & thyroglossal procedures w/o CC/MCC	1.1828	1.4
628	S*	Other endocrine, nutrit & metab O.R. proc w MCC	3.6794	7.4
629	S*	Other endocrine, nutrit & metab O.R. proc w CC	2.3453	6.1
630	S*	Other endocrine, nutrit & metab O.R. proc w/o CC/MCC	1.4093	2.3
637	M*	Diabetes w MCC	1.3766	3.8
638	M*	Diabetes w CC	0.8794	2.9
639	M*	Diabetes w/o CC/MCC	0.6096	2.1
640	M*	Misc disorders of nutrition, metab, fluids/electrolytes w MCC	1.2308	3.3
641	M*	Misc disorders of nutrition, metab, fluids/electrolytes w/o MCC	0.7542	2.6
642	M	Inborn and other disorders of metabolism	1.2898	3.3
643	M*	Endocrine disorders w MCC	1.6677	5.0
644	M*	Endocrine disorders w CC	1.0198	3.5
645	M*	Endocrine disorders w/o CC/MCC	0.7686	2.7
650	S	Kidney Transplant with Hemodialysis with MCC	4.5207	6.8
651	S	Kidney Transplant with Hemodialysis without MCC	3.6984	6.0
652	S	Kidney transplant	3.1851	4.7
653	S*	Major bladder procedures w MCC	5.4592	10.2

654	S*	Major bladder procedures w CC	2.9028	5.6
655	S*	Major bladder procedures w/o CC/MCC	2.0803	3.6
656	S	Kidney & ureter procedures for neoplasm w MCC	3.2850	5.6
657	S	Kidney & ureter procedures for neoplasm w CC	1.9347	3.2
658	S	Kidney & ureter procedures for neoplasm w/o CC/MCC	1.5779	2.1
659	S*	Kidney & ureter procedures for non-neoplasm w MCC	2.6664	5.9
660	S*	Kidney & ureter procedures for non-neoplasm w CC	1.4431	3.1
661	S*	Kidney & ureter procedures for non-neoplasm w/o CC/MCC	1.0637	1.9
662	S	Minor bladder procedures w MCC	2.9373	6.9
663	S	Minor bladder procedures w CC	1.5995	3.7
664	S	Minor bladder procedures w/o CC/MCC	1.1838	1.9
665	S	Prostatectomy w MCC	3.0417	7.6
666	S	Prostatectomy w CC	1.7397	4.0
667	S	Prostatectomy w/o CC/MCC	0.9975	2.0
668	S	Transurethral procedures w MCC	2.8063	7.1
669	S	Transurethral procedures w CC	1.5635	3.8
670	S	Transurethral procedures w/o CC/MCC	0.9785	2.1
671	S	Urethral procedures w CC/MCC	1.7813	3.9
672	S	Urethral procedures w/o CC/MCC	1.1504	1.6
673	S	Other kidney & urinary tract procedures w MCC	3.4683	7.7
674	S	Other kidney & urinary tract procedures w CC	2.3832	5.9
675	S	Other kidney & urinary tract procedures w/o CC/MCC	1.7547	2.7

682	M*	Renal failure *w MCC*	1.4727	4.3
683	M*	Renal failure *w CC*	0.8793	3.1
684	M*	Renal failure *w/o CC/MCC*	0.6079	2.2
686	M	Kidney & urinary tract neoplasms *w MCC*	1.8753	5.0
687	M	Kidney & urinary tract neoplasms *w CC*	1.0501	3.3
688	M	Kidney & urinary tract neoplasms *w/o CC/MCC*	0.6858	1.9
689	M*	Kidney & urinary tract infections *w MCC*	1.1142	3.8
690	M*	Kidney & urinary tract infections *w/o MCC*	0.7940	2.9
693	M	Urinary stones *w MCC*	1.3355	3.7
694	M	Urinary stones *w/o MCC*	0.7712	2.1
695	M	Kidney & urinary tract signs & symptoms *w MCC*	1.1377	3.6
696	M	Kidney & urinary tract signs & symptoms *w/o MCC*	0.6919	2.3
697	M	Urethral stricture	0.9993	2.8
698	M*	Other kidney & urinary tract diagnoses *w MCC*	1.6106	4.7
699	M*	Other kidney & urinary tract diagnoses *w CC*	1.0270	3.3
700	M*	Other kidney & urinary tract diagnoses *w/o CC/MCC*	0.7465	2.4
707	S	Major male pelvic procedures *w CC/MCC*	1.9222	2.5
708	S	Major male pelvic procedures *w/o CC/MCC*	1.4912	1.4
709	S	Penis procedures *w CC/MCC*	2.3159	4.0
710	S	Penis procedures *w/o CC/MCC*	1.6016	1.7
711	S	Testes procedures *w CC/MCC*	2.1316	5.3
712	S	Testes procedures *w/o CC/MCC*	1.0600	2.5

713	S	Transurethral prostatectomy w CC/MCC	1.4934	2.8
714	S	Transurethral prostatectomy w/o CC/MCC	0.9288	1.6
715	S	Other male reproductive system O.R. proc for malignancy w CC/MCC	2.0216	5.0
716	S	Other male reproductive system O.R. proc for malignancy w/o CC/MCC	1.2758	1.4
717	S	Other male reproductive system O.R. proc exc malignancy w CC/MCC	1.8006	3.7
718	S	Other male reproductive system O.R. proc exc malignancy w/o CC/MCC	1.2346	2.2
722	M	Malignancy, male reproductive system w MCC	1.7126	5.1
723	M	Malignancy, male reproductive system w CC	1.0919	3.5
724	M	Malignancy, male reproductive system w/o CC/MCC	0.6481	1.8
725	M	Benign prostatic hypertrophy w MCC	1.2855	4.0
726	M	Benign prostatic hypertrophy w/o MCC	0.7447	2.5
727	M	Inflammation of the male reproductive system w MCC	1.4210	4.4
728	M	Inflammation of the male reproductive system w/o MCC	0.8057	3.0
729	M	Other male reproductive system diagnoses w CC/MCC	1.0075	3.1
730	M	Other male reproductive system diagnoses w/o CC/MCC	0.5689	1.8
734	S	Pelvic evisceration, rad hysterectomy & rad vulvectomy w CC/MCC	2.2243	3.5
735	S	Pelvic evisceration, rad hysterectomy & rad vulvectomy w/o CC/MCC	1.4136	1.7
736	S	Uterine & adnexa proc for ovarian or adnexal malignancy w MCC	4.2607	8.4
737	S	Uterine & adnexa proc for ovarian or adnexal malignancy w CC	2.0581	4.2
738	S	Uterine & adnexa proc for ovarian or adnexal malignancy w/o CC/MCC	1.4759	2.6
739	S	Uterine, adnexa proc for non-ovarian/adnexal malig w MCC	3.8240	6.6
740	S	Uterine, adnexa proc for non-ovarian/adnexal malig w CC	1.8016	2.8

333

741	S	Uterine, adnexa proc for non-ovarian/adnexal malig w/o CC/MCC	1.2799	1.6
742	S	Uterine & adnexa proc for non-malignancy w CC/MCC	1.7181	2.8
743	S	Uterine & adnexa proc for non-malignancy w/o CC/MCC	1.1328	1.7
744	S	D&C, conization, laparoscopy & tubal interruption w CC/MCC	1.7954	4.4
745	S	D&C, conization, laparoscopy & tubal interruption w/o CC/MCC	1.1700	2.2
746	S	Vagina, cervix & vulva procedures w CC/MCC	1.6115	3.2
747	S	Vagina, cervix & vulva procedures w/o CC/MCC	0.9391	1.5
748	S	Female reproductive system reconstructive procedures	1.3476	1.6
749	S	Other female reproductive system O.R. procedures w CC/MCC	2.7138	5.6
750	S	Other female reproductive system O.R. procedures w/o CC/MCC	1.4638	2.3
754	M	Malignancy, female reproductive system w MCC	1.8262	5.0
755	M	Malignancy, female reproductive system w CC	1.1293	3.3
756	M	Malignancy, female reproductive system w/o CC/MCC	0.9184	2.1
757	M	Infections, female reproductive system w MCC	1.5247	4.7
758	M	Infections, female reproductive system w CC	0.9697	3.6
759	M	Infections, female reproductive system w/o CC/MCC	0.6834	2.7
760	M	Menstrual & other female reproductive system disorders w CC/MCC	0.9201	2.6
761	M	Menstrual & other female reproductive system disorders w/o CC/MCC	0.5908	1.8
768	S	Vaginal delivery w O.R. proc except steril &/or D&C	1.1696	3.1
769	S	Postpartum & post abortion diagnoses w O.R. procedure	1.6176	2.9
770	S	Abortion w D&C, aspiration curettage or hysterotomy	0.8898	1.8
776	M	Postpartum & post abortion diagnoses w/o O.R. procedure	0.7745	2.5

779	M	Abortion w/o D&C	1.0590	2.0
783	S	Cesarean section w sterilization w MCC	1.8749	4.8
784	S	Cesarean section w sterilization w CC	1.0959	3.3
785	S	Cesarean section w sterilization w/o CC/MCC	0.9168	2.7
786	S	Cesarean section w/o sterilization w MCC	1.5944	4.3
787	S	Cesarean section w/o sterilization w CC	1.0644	3.5
788	S	Cesarean section w/o sterilization w/o CC/MCC	0.8874	3.0
789	M	Neonates, died or transferred to another acute care facility	1.7200	1.8
790	M	Extreme immaturity or respiratory distress syndrome, neonate	5.6721	17.9
791	M	Prematurity w major problems	3.8738	13.3
792	M	Prematurity w/o major problems	2.3374	8.6
793	M	Full term neonate w major problems	3.9792	4.7
794	M	Neonate w other significant problems	1.4084	3.4
795	M	Normal newborn	0.1907	3.1
796	S	Vaginal delivery w sterilization/D&C w MCC	1.0708	3.6
797	S	Vaginal delivery w sterilization/D&C w CC	0.9194	2.4
798	S	Vaginal delivery w sterilization/D&C w/o CC/MCC	0.8275	2.1
799	S	Splenectomy w MCC	5.1474	7.8
800	S	Splenectomy w CC	2.9539	5.0
801	S	Splenectomy w/o CC/MCC	1.6840	2.6
802	S	Other O.R. proc of the blood & blood forming organs w MCC	3.7117	7.5
803	S	Other O.R. proc of the blood & blood forming organs w CC	1.8865	3.9

MS-DRG TABLE

804	S	Other O.R. proc of the blood & blood forming organs w/o CC/MCC	1.3659	2.0
805	M	Vaginal delivery w/o sterilization/D&C w MCC	1.0299	2.9
806	M	Vaginal delivery w/o sterilization/D&C w CC	0.7346	2.3
807	M	Vaginal delivery w/o sterilization/D&C w w/o CC/MCC	0.6423	2.1
808	M	Major hematol/immun diag exc sickle cell crisis & coagul w MCC	2.1858	5.4
809	M	Major hematol/immun diag exc sickle cell crisis & coagul w CC	1.2234	3.5
810	M	Major hematol/immun diag exc sickle cell crisis & coagul w/o CC/MCC	0.9617	2.5
811	M	Red blood cell disorders w MCC	1.3793	3.6
812	M	Red blood cell disorders w/o MCC	0.8803	2.7
813	M	Coagulation disorders	1.5451	3.6
814	M	Reticuloendothelial & immunity disorders w MCC	1.8917	4.5
815	M	Reticuloendothelial & immunity disorders w CC	0.9934	2.9
816	M	Reticuloendothelial & immunity disorders w/o CC/MCC	0.6611	2.2
817	S	Other antepartum diagnoses w O.R. procedure w MCC	2.3068	4.1
818	S	Other antepartum diagnoses w O.R. procedure w CC	1.3598	3.0
819	S	Other antepartum diagnoses w O.R. procedure w/o CC/MCC	0.9872	1.7
820	S	Lymphoma & leukemia w major O.R. procedure w MCC	5.6917	10.6
821	S	Lymphoma & leukemia w major O.R. procedure w CC	2.1552	3.7
822	S	Lymphoma & leukemia w major O.R. procedure w/o CC/MCC	1.2515	1.8
823	S	Lymphoma & non-acute leukemia w other O.R. proc w MCC	4.5018	10.3
824	S	Lymphoma & non-acute leukemia w other O.R. proc w CC	2.3644	5.3
825	S	Lymphoma & non-acute leukemia w other O.R. proc w/o CC/MCC	1.4015	2.4

826	S	Myeloprolif disord or poorly diff neopl *w maj O.R. proc w MCC*	5.0445	9.9
827	S	Myeloprolif disord or poorly diff neopl *w maj O.R. proc w CC*	2.5006	4.9
828	S	Myeloprolif disord or poorly diff neopl *w maj O.R. proc w/o CC/MCC*	1.6740	2.8
829	S	Myeloprolif disord or poorly diff neopl *w other proc w CC/MCC*	3.2084	6.2
830	S	Myeloprolif disord or poorly diff neopl *w other proc w/o CC/MCC*	1.4820	2.3
831	M	Other antepartum diagnoses *w/o O.R. procedure w MCC*	1.1218	3.4
832	M	Other antepartum diagnoses *w/o O.R. procedure w CC*	0.7783	2.5
833	M	Other antepartum diagnoses *w/o O.R. procedure w/o CC/MCC*	0.5370	1.9
834	M	Acute leukemia *w/o major O.R. procedure w MCC*	6.0522	10.0
835	M	Acute leukemia *w/o major O.R. procedure w CC*	2.1137	4.2
836	M	Acute leukemia *w/o major O.R. procedure w/o CC/MCC*	1.1735	2.7
837	M	Chemo *w acute leukemia as sdx or w high dose chemo agent w MCC*	5.6993	11.5
838	M	Chemo *w acute leukemia as sdx w CC or high dose chemo agent*	2.2602	5.5
839	M	Chemo *w acute leukemia as sdx w/o CC/MCC*	1.4872	4.4
840	M*	Lymphoma & non-acute leukemia *w MCC*	3.2205	6.7
841	M*	Lymphoma & non-acute leukemia *w CC*	1.6216	4.0
842	M*	Lymphoma & non-acute leukemia *w/o CC/MCC*	1.0970	2.8
843	M	Other myeloprolif dis or poorly diff neopl diag *w MCC*	1.9076	5.3
844	M	Other myeloprolif dis or poorly diff neopl diag *w CC*	1.1842	3.6
845	M	Other myeloprolif dis or poorly diff neopl diag *w/o CC/MCC*	0.8489	2.6
846	M	Chemotherapy *w/o acute leukemia as secondary diagnosis w MCC*	2.6729	5.9
847	M	Chemotherapy *w/o acute leukemia as secondary diagnosis w CC*	1.3361	3.6

848	M	Chemotherapy *w/o acute leukemia as secondary diagnosis w/o CC/MCC*	1.0323	3.0
849	M	Radiotherapy	2.4936	6.2
853	S*	Infectious & parasitic diseases *w O.R. procedure w MCC*	4.9678	9.6
854	S*	Infectious & parasitic diseases *w O.R. procedure w CC*	2.1222	5.3
855	S*	Infectious & parasitic diseases *w O.R. procedure w/o CC/MCC*	1.5198	3.3
856	S*	Postoperative or post-traumatic infections *w O.R. proc w MCC*	4.6639	9.2
857	S*	Postoperative or post-traumatic infections *w O.R. proc w CC*	2.1024	5.4
858	S*	Postoperative or post-traumatic infections *w O.R. proc w/o CC/MCC*	1.3596	3.5
862	M*	Postoperative & post-traumatic infections *w MCC*	1.8967	5.0
863	M*	Postoperative & post-traumatic infections *w/o MCC*	1.0114	3.5
864	M	Fever and inflammatory conditions	0.8765	2.7
865	M	Viral illness *w MCC*	1.4778	3.9
866	M	Viral illness *w/o MCC*	0.8390	2.7
867	M*	Other infectious & parasitic diseases diagnoses *w MCC*	2.2371	5.5
868	M*	Other infectious & parasitic diseases diagnoses *w CC*	1.0660	3.5
869	M*	Other infectious & parasitic diseases diagnoses *w/o CC/MCC*	0.7285	2.5
870	M*	Septicemia or severe sepsis *w MV >96 hours*	6.4390	12.4
871	M*	Septicemia or severe sepsis *w/o MV >96 hours w MCC*	1.8722	4.8
872	M*	Septicemia or severe sepsis *w/o MV >96 hours w/o MCC*	1.0263	3.5
876	S	O.R. procedure *w principal diagnoses of mental illness*	3.2680	7.0
880	M	Acute adjustment reaction & psychosocial dysfunction	0.8645	2.6
881	M	Depressive neuroses	0.8020	3.9

882	M	Neuroses except depressive	0.8236	3.2
883	M	Disorders of personality & impulse control	1.5818	5.1
884	M*	Organic disturbances & intellectual disability	1.4473	4.5
885	M	Psychoses	1.2394	5.9
886	M	Behavioral & developmental disorders	1.2237	4.3
887	M	Other mental disorder diagnoses	1.0798	3.0
894	M	Alcohol/drug abuse or dependence, left AMA	0.5490	2.0
895	M	Alcohol/drug abuse or dependence *w rehabilitation therapy*	1.5992	8.9
896	M*	Alcohol/drug abuse or dependence *w/o rehabilitation therapy w MCC*	1.7803	4.9
897	M*	Alcohol/drug abuse or dependence *w/o rehabilitation therapy w/o MCC*	0.8270	3.4
901	S	Wound debridements for injuries *w MCC*	4.2687	8.8
902	S	Wound debridements for injuries *w CC*	1.9643	4.8
903	S	Wound debridements for injuries *w/o CC/MCC*	1.1353	2.6
904	S	Skin grafts for injuries *w CC/MCC*	3.7270	7.1
905	S	Skin grafts for injuries *w/o CC/MCC*	1.6500	3.3
906	S	Hand procedures for injuries	1.8038	2.8
907	S*	Other O.R. procedures for injuries *w MCC*	3.9482	6.8
908	S*	Other O.R. procedures for injuries *w CC*	2.0504	3.9
909	S*	Other O.R. procedures for injuries *w/o CC/MCC*	1.3710	2.4
913	M	Traumatic injury *w MCC*	1.6386	3.7
914	M	Traumatic injury *w/o MCC*	0.8869	2.5
915	M	Allergic reactions *w MCC*	1.6995	3.7

916	M	Allergic reactions w/o MCC	0.6584	1.8
917	M*	Poisoning & toxic effects of drugs w MCC	1.4785	3.5
918	M*	Poisoning & toxic effects of drugs w/o MCC	0.7916	2.3
919	M	Complications of treatment w MCC	1.8441	4.3
920	M	Complications of treatment w CC	1.0246	2.9
921	M	Complications of treatment w/o CC/MCC	0.6979	2.1
922	M	Other injury, poisoning & toxic effect diag w MCC	1.5882	4.1
923	M	Other injury, poisoning & toxic effect diag w/o MCC	0.9398	2.7
927	S	Extensive burns or full thickness burns w MV >96 hrs w skin graft	21.0913	26.0
928	S	Full thickness burn w skin graft or inhal inj w CC/MCC	6.5316	11.7
929	S	Full thickness burn w skin graft or inhal inj w/o CC/MCC	3.0139	5.9
933	M	Extensive burns or full thickness burns w MV >96 hrs w/o skin graft	2.2629	2.4
934	M	Full thickness burn w/o skin graft or inhal inj	1.9409	4.3
935	M	Non-extensive burns	1.9329	3.6
939	S	O.R. proc w diagnoses of other contact w health services w MCC	3.3746	6.6
940	S	O.R. proc w diagnoses of other contact w health services w CC	2.2209	3.5
941	S	O.R. proc w diagnoses of other contact w health services w/o CC/MCC	1.9231	2.2
945	M*	Rehabilitation w CC/MCC	1.4819	5.0
946	M*	Rehabilitation w/o CC/MCC	1.1262	3.2
947	M*	Signs & symptoms w MCC	1.1940	3.5
948	M*	Signs & symptoms w/o MCC	0.7871	2.6
949	M	Aftercare w CC/MCC	1.1099	4.3

950	M	Aftercare *w/o CC/MCC*	0.7402	3.0
951	M	Other factors influencing health status	0.5596	1.8
955	S	Craniotomy for multiple significant trauma	6.2893	7.3
956	S*	Limb reattachment, hip & femur proc for multiple significant trauma	3.8500	6.0
957	S	Other O.R. procedures for multiple significant trauma *w MCC*	7.4209	9.1
958	S	Other O.R. procedures for multiple significant trauma *w CC*	4.2057	6.7
959	S	Other O.R. procedures for multiple significant trauma *w/o CC/MCC*	2.7361	4.2
963	M	Other multiple significant trauma *w MCC*	2.7299	5.2
964	M	Other multiple significant trauma *w CC*	1.4918	3.9
965	M	Other multiple significant trauma *w/o CC/MCC*	0.9125	2.6
969	S	HIV with extensive O.R. procedure *w MCC*	5.8519	11.1
970	S	HIV with extensive O.R. procedure *w/o MCC*	2.9887	6.6
974	M	HIV with major related condition *w MCC*	2.6905	6.3
975	M	HIV with major related condition *w CC*	1.2821	4.0
976	M	HIV with major related condition *w/o CC/MCC*	0.9496	3.0
977	M	*HIV w or w/o other related condition*	1.3243	3.6
981	S*	Extensive O.R. procedure unrelated to principal diagnosis *w MCC*	4.6145	8.4
982	S*	Extensive O.R. procedure unrelated to principal diagnosis *w CC*	2.5366	4.6
983	S*	Extensive O.R. procedure unrelated to principal diagnosis *w/o CC/MCC*	1.6523	2.3
987	S*	Non-extensive O.R. proc unrelated to principal diagnosis *w MCC*	3.2759	7.7
988	S*	Non-extensive O.R. proc unrelated to principal diagnosis *w CC*	1.7064	4.3
989	S*	Non-extensive O.R. proc unrelated to principal diagnosis *w/o CC/MCC*	1.1236	2.3